NEUROPLASTICITY

Simple Strategies to Better Manage Your Life

(Newest Guide to Working Brain Plasticity and Rewiring Your Brain)

Joseph Galant

Published By Regina Loviusher

Joseph Galante

All Rights Reserved

Neuroplasticity: Simple Strategies to Better Manage Your Life (Newest Guide to Working Brain Plasticity and Rewiring Your Brain)

ISBN 978-1-77485-373-3

Legal & Disclaimer

The information contained in this book is not designed to replace or take the place of any form of medicine or professional medical advice. The information in this book has been provided for educational and entertainment purposes only.

The information contained in this book has been compiled from sources deemed reliable, and it is accurate to the best of the Author's knowledge; however, the Author cannot guarantee its accuracy and validity and cannot be held liable for any errors or omissions. Changes are periodically made to this book. You must consult your doctor or get professional medical advice before using any of the suggested remedies, techniques, or information in this book.

Table of Contents

Introduction

The chapters that follow will explain the things you need to be aware of before you begin making use of mental models to meet your personal needs. There are plenty of different techniques for managing time and strategies you could test, and a lot are effective however if you are looking to cut down on the time required to make your decisions, make sure that you are making the best choices and in the end, make life more manageable. This guidebook will spend some time discussing the different mental models and how they are going help you, and the various types of mental models you can apply in accordance with the problems you'd like to accomplish.

For the first part of this guidebook we will explore the mental models that are about. This will help us understand the purpose behind these models and the advantages that they provide. It is also possible to examine the power of these mental models and the top mental models that can be utilized in conjunction with many of the other subjects we'll examine in this guidebook.

Once we've got the basic mental models in place and ready for use and ready to go, we can look into the practical applications of these mental models and how to make use of them in a variety of different personality types and aspects also. It is evident they are effective great for making choices, for entrepreneurs and other parts of running a business. They are also great for those who are studying and curious and can help you develop your parenting skills for critical thinkers as well as educators, as well as those who want to develop their own personal growth. In these areas we will examine more deeply the mental models and how you can use them throughout your life.

In order to conclude this book, we're going to look at various case studies that deal with the mental models. These can help us understand how the mental models the real world, which means that we are not just working from theories, but can actually understand the specific ways in which these mental models are utilized!

A significant amount of time and effort could be spent thinking about things and making choices The longer we think about those thoughts the more lost we are. Mental models assist us to clear the confusion by giving us a handful of the strategies are needed to make things work. If you're looking to know more about mental models and how they function ensure you go through this book to get you started.

There are a lot of books on the subject available out there, so thanks to everyone who chose this book! We have made every effort to ensure it's packed with as much valuable information as is possible. Please take advantage of it!

Chapter 1: Functional Brain

The gut and the brain are inextricably linked. We feel 'gut-felt regarding a person or event, and we feel butterflies in our stomachs when something thrilling occurs. Neuroscientists have been more aware that the gut can contain crucial information about the brain's function.

The gut has the appearance of a miniature brain, an extensive network of neurons known as"the enteric nervous system. The brain and the enteric nerve system communicate together, and the communications line that connects the two is commonly referred to as the gut brain axis.

What can we do to improve the microbiome in our gut?

I imagine the micro biome in the same way as the diverse soils that plants thrive in on. Some plants thrive in compost that is rich in nutrients, however they will not thrive in a sandy, dry soil. Western diets, specifically ones with low levels of fiber, may have diminished the diversity of microbiota over time. Contrarily, traditional food items rich in fiber and lower in fat and sugar can boost the diversity of microbiome

What could we be doing to make sure the microbiome of our body is supportive of our well-being?

Researchers have suggested that the variety and functions of microbiome are influenced by your genetic background as well as external factors, such as the method of delivery you received at birth and the manner in which you exercise. The most significant factor in the composition and the activity of the microbiome in your gut is your diet which accounts for about 78.6 percent of variances in the total microbiota of your gut.

We can affect the population of microbes in our gut in our gut by creating an friendly to them through eating prebiotic and probiotic foods.

Probiotics are food or dietary supplements that contain specific beneficial microbes for the gut (such as Lactobacillus and Bifid bacteria) to boost the growth of microorganisms within the digestive tract.

Probiotic-rich food items include live yogurt and kombucha. Kamahi and fermented veggies like sauerkraut.

Prebiotics are food items that encourage the development of healthy bacteria. I consider them to be an nutrient-rich fertilizer which helps plants to grow. Prebiotic-rich food items include bananas, wheat, onions, flaxseeds, wheat legumes, leaves of green, e.g., spinach, broccoli, kale, and more. Fermented foods are full of bacteria that support digestion and are prebiotic. Live bacteria have already been working.

The brain-gut-micro biome is an axis

Another key player is in the gut-brain interaction. The intestines in our body are home to an community of microbes which regulate digestion, fight off pathogens, and regulate neurotransmitter and hormone production. The whole of these microbes is referred to as the 'gut microbiome'. The average person has 1.5 kilograms of bacteria within their guts - comparable to the size that the human brain weighs! Gut bacteria also make neurotransmitters g-aminobutyric acid (GABA) serotonin dopamine and acetylcholine.Gut bacteria communicate with the enteric nervous system as well as the brain, however the exact mechanism of communication is not known. Researchers refer to it as 'black box connectivity.' The possible routes of communication are the use of hormones and immune signaling molecules metabolic pathways, and the mysterious nerve.

The gut-brain superhighway

Gut communication is conducted with the brain through hormones that are released into the bloodstream that travel across the blood-brain-brain barrier, regulating our craving to eat. For instance stomach hormones ghrelin alerts us when we're hungry . Likewise, other hormones, like the glucagon-like one can influence satiety and tell us when we're hungry. These hormones affect the reward-signaling neural pathways in the brain, which explains the reason why foods taste better when we're hungry.

The gut also produces neurotransmitters, which are proteins that neurons utilize to talk to synapses. One of these neurotransmitters is serotonin. About 80% of body's total serotonin production is in the gut. The remaining is made within the nerve system. Within the stomach enterochromaffin cells that line the stomach's wall make and produce serotonin, where it plays a crucial part in controlling the peristalsis waves-like contractions of the intestinal walls that push food down in the digestive tract. Certain neurons of the digestive nervous system produce and utilize serotonin as neurotransmitters.

Note! The gut isn't the brain's "serotonin production facility.' Neurons in the brain produce their neurotransmitters. Additionally, serotonin that is secreted in the gut and other neurotransmitters are not able to traverse the blood-brain-barrier, which means it's unlikely that gut serotonin will directly influences brain function via the bloodstream.

How can gut bugs communicate in the mind?

The gut creates an environment where bacteria can ferment digested foods into all sorts of chemical and molecule which inform the brain about our nutritional status. As we discussed in the previous blog, the microbiome transmits information to the brain via channels like obscure nerve, immune, and hormone systems, as well as through the bioactive microbial metabolites released into bloodstreams.

Short-chain fats (SCFAs) are the metabolites created in the gut via microbiological fermentation of diet fibers along with complex carbohydrates. They can pass through the blood-brain barrier and influence the brain's activity to regulate the appetite and intake of food. Within the brain SCFAs can protect neurons.

One of these SCFAs is butyric acid , also known as butyrate. Butyrate is an anti-inflammatory substance within the brain and gut , and it reduces the levels of toxic neurotoxic toxins that could harm neurons. It also strengthens the blood-brain-barrier by making connections more secure between cells that prevent harmful toxins from getting into the brain and causing neuron-damaging inflammation. A damaged blood-brain barrier frequently seen in obese people and neurodegenerative diseases like Alzheimer's disease. Butyrate can also increase the production of the molecules crucial for neuroplasticity such as the brain-derived neurotropic factors (BDNF). The increased levels of BDNF can lead to improved performance in memory tests on lab rats. Researchers have discovered that eating unhealthy diet can reduce SCFA levels, which is why it is crucial to eat an appropriate diet to ensure the optimal functioning of your brain.

Squeaky clean mice

The majority of microbiome research conducted to date has utilized mice that are germ-free and raised in sterilized conditions. Germ-free mice are born through Caesarean section, thus preventing transmission of bacteria to their mother. They are raised in isolation units that are sterile, they eat clean water and food, and breathe air filtered. Mice that are free of germs provide an uncluttered canvas for their microbiome in the gut.

Fecal microbiome transplants FMTs, which are poo transplants in mice free of germs permit researchers to investigate the ways in which a particular microbiome in the gut can alter the function of the brain. For instance, after receiving the poo, germ-free mice take on the behavior characteristics similar to the mice that donated the poo. A study found that mice receiving FMTs from stressed mice were more anxious in unfamiliar environmentsin essence, passing on nervousness from their pet's. Contrastingly, mice that were germ-free that received FMTs from interested and curious mice were less nervous when confronted with unfamiliar situations.

These studies suggest that the presence and composition of the gut micro biota, which transmits signals to the brain through the gut-brain-axis which alters the emotions of rodents.

It is important to know that mice that are free of germs are not normal mice. They are raised in artificial environments that resemble bubbles without microorganisms to develop the immune system. They have a distinct behavior from normal lab mice, specifically, stress-related reactions as well as social reactions.

Could we help balance our brains with bacteria?

Modifying the microbiome with FMTs could alter the brain's chemical makeup. Studies in humans have suggested that FMTs might have therapeutic potential in the treatment of the chronic fatigue syndrome, autism and MS, but it is necessary to conduct more research. There is a well-respected gap between the research of rodents in neuroscience and its applications in humans.

My next article, I'll explain how scientists manipulate the microbiome with the help of "psychobiotics" to treat mood disorders , and also making use of probiotics as well as prebiotics to boost brain health.

Our intestines house an ecosystem that is comprised of billions of microbes that include bacteria as well as viruses, phages protests, fungi and Nematodes. Most prevalent are bacteria from the families of Formicates as well as Bacteriodetes. In my previous blog, the collective group of these microbes that live in the intestines constitutes the gut micro biome.'

This blog will examine the gut microbiome from the point of view in obesity-related research. The changes in the gut microbiome are associated with a range of health states , including obesity. Obesity-related microbes can influence insulin resistance inflammation, metabolism, fat deposition and appetite. The gut microbiome is now a focus for new therapies to treat obesity.

What is the microbiome's role in our health? impact our well-being?

The gut microbiome responds to the environment around it, and also to the food we consume. Healthy and unhealthy diets influence the microbiome, including what species dominate.

In other words eating a diet that is loaded with sugar and saturated fat can alter the balance between good bacteriatericides and the 'bad' cutes bacteria. Formicates are required to digest fats, and the diet high in fats encourages the population to grow and, in turn, leads to weight growth. Bacteriodetes digest fiber soluble which is why people who consume high-fiber foods have higher levels of Bacteriodetes than formicates.

Researchers studying mice that are germ-free who lack microbes in their guts and found that an alteration in how balance was maintained among Bacteriodetes and formicates determined the extent to which mice were obese or lean. become. The propensity to be obese or leanness may be transmitted from mouse to mouse through gut microbes on their own.

The brain controls the appetite, feeding habits, and balance of energy, and even though the gut microbiome is a factor in obesity and metabolic disorders such as diabetes, the specific mechanism behind this connection is not clear. The connection between the microbiome and the prevalence of obesity in humans can be described as "weak."

Chapter 2: Human Memory - History And Development Of Analysis

From the time of ancient times, philosophers, scholars and rhetoricians have used the human brain to better understand its intricate functions. They utilized their scarce resources, observed their subjects, and then write about their findings. David Hartley, the 18th century English philosopher, presented his theories on the function of the brain. He proposed that the memory stored in the nerve system can retrieve the information through its concealed motions.It was a flawed theory, basic in its principle but is still the most comprehensive research on human memory.

Beyond that the scope of this article, we have a treatise written by Aristotle in his 'On the Soul', in which the human brain is described as a 'blank sheet. ' He further hypothesized, people are born with a 'blank brain' without any knowledge and filled with information on a later stage of life, which are sum up of their experiences.Aristotle's theory considered as an acceptable format of explanations until the time David Hartley released his new findings.The conclusions of Aristotle relate memory something similar to making an impression on a wax - "storehouse metaphor."

The earliest studies of brain and memory were based on assumptionsuntil 1880. In 1890. Herman Ebbinghaus, a German philosopher, and William James; an American psychologist, published their findings in scientific journals on human memory. According to the old assumptions that brains have two parts that are the natural memory and the artificial memory.' The natural memory refers to activities that require you to recall daily things that are used on a daily basis. Artificial memory is used to the process of learning that is trained, that makes use of Mnemonic methods, when you need to complete difficult tasks using a the process of memory training.

Mnemonics are methods used to help you recall information that is difficult to remember.Ancient Romans practiced, various methods for memorization. During the period of Quintilian and Cicero who did an extensive study of memory processes and memorization techniques, they developed a method of memorization, "the Art of Memory" sometimes referred to as the'method' of loci. "Mind palace technique" or "memory palace technique' are two names that can be used to describe the loci methods that use visual patterns to boost the memory using spatial memory. The technique involves recalling the surroundings, in which the incident took place and assisting in retrieving the relevant information.

Turning Point Towards Modern Psychology:

The research that were discovered by Cicero and Quintilian were extensively utilized by a variety of Roman scholars. Some of the most prominent rhetoricians included Matteo Ricci and Giordano Bruno. Despite all the efforts made by prominent researchers and philosophers, the credit for the modern psychology's founders is given directly to William James, the famous American psychologist, and Wilhelm Maximilian Wundt of Germany who was a physiologist and physician. Their groundbreaking research papers that were published between 1870 and 1880, formed the foundational pillars of modern psychology. William James discussed the possibility of neural plasticity throughout his work "The The Principles of Psychology."

The same time in 1881, a contemporary French psychologists speculated on the possible causes of amnesia, more commonly referred to as Ribot's Law.Although the results aren't perfect however, they are the most important work to reveal secrets that relates to amnesia.Amnesia is a state in which people forget what they have done or are unable to remember things because of various causes.

The first method of scientific research:

It was in 1880 that we were given the first scientific method developed in the form of Herman Ebbinghaus, pioneer of the research into memory and well-known for his work "Forgetting Curve and Spacing Effect." He classified memory into sensory, long-term and short-term that has relevance to now.He experimented by using nonsense syllables, and linking them to the sense of words and was the key to creating "Forgetting Curve and Spacing Effect."

The brain stores memories:

The study of cognitive psychology of Sir Frederick Bartlett, who was a British psychologist, proposed the concept of the brain's complex actions and the capacity to'recall events from 1930. His work greatly contributed to shedding more light on memory storage and memory. Before the research by Sir Frederick Bartlett, another German biologist Richard Semon identified the possibilities and explained that experience leaves physical marks on specific neurons in the brain.He described the problem as an engram.'

The decade of the nineties gave a lot of information about the brain and memory activities.Extensive study by Karl Spencer Lashley, a well-known US psychologist conducted on rats by placing artificial mazes to determine the exact location where memories or engrams that form within the brain.Engram is a scenario which causes permanent changes in the brain, which is believed to be the main reason behind that there is memory.After an uninterrupted 25 years of research and experiments, around 1950, Karl Spencer Lashley published his study, asserting that memories do not connect in a particular part of the brain. Instead it is a fusion of the whole cortex.

The research on flashback are also a crucial aspect of psychology, in which researchers like the Canadian neurosurgeon Wilder Penfield had put a significant contribution in 1950.Similarly the link between neurons as well as the process of memories are encoded was discovered when neurons interacted to each other, as proposed in the work of Donald Hebb, a Canadian psychologist who conducted extensive study. The results of his research are known as Hebb's Rule which remains an effective theory in the present today.Hebb's theory has the scientific backing of Eric Kandel's work on sea slugs , which confirms the molecular changes and fluctuations in neurotransmitters throughout the process of learning.

Coding, storage and retrieval:

The encoding, storage, and retrieval are the three crucial brain processes and psychologist that are put to use with various theories and hypotheses to investigate the subject.We may witness an enormous leap in the field of memory during the 1960's, and the research was referred to"cognitive revolution. "cognitive revolution. "There are a lot of papers written about short-term memories, sensorimotor memory and long-term memory as well as working memory.Out of them, the book written by George Miller on short-term memory is quite impressive, and is proof of the limitations in short-term memory.

The multi-store model of memory that includes short-term memory, sensory memory , and long-term memory, published by Richard Atkinson and Richard Shiffrin in 1968 was The Magna Carta of memory-related study for an extended periodof time, right up to the 'levels process' model was published in 1972 by Fergus Craik and Robert Lockhart in 1972.

Working memory

in 1974, a novel hypothesis on the concept of working (short-term) memory" was proposed in 1974 by Alan Baddeley and Graham Hitch with the main elements that were based on the work of the collective of the visuospatial pencil, central executiveas well as the phonological loops as a method to encoding.We must remember that encoding is the main procedure for creating the ability to create a new memory.The whole concept of working memory was designed to determine the function of the brain to store the information that is temporary at any point of need, confirming the existence of a "scratch-pad" that acts as the Post-it note inside the brain.

False memories are the nature:

From the 70s, onwards, neuropsychology saw a flood of papers. And out of them the papers about the 'nature of false memories misinformation effect, false memories, and memory biases' by Elisabeth Loftus were of great importance. The papers on memory for long-term as well as episodic memory by Endel Tulving during the years 1970-1972 were widely debated within the scientific community and held great significance in the understanding of the nature of memory.

The paper he wrote on the 'encoding the principle of specificity,' which was which was published in the year 1983, was a highly acclaimed research paper on memory function.

Cognitive neuroscience:

The current research into human memory includes two distinct sections, the cognitive and neuroscience that are deeply interconnected and is referred to as cognition neuroscience. Between 1980 and 1990, there were numerous research papers that were published in the field of cognitive neuroscience. The most well-known works included the 'Search for Associative Memory (SAM) model released in 1981 as a collaborative study of Richard Shiffrin and Jerome Raaijmaker. Other notable works include the joint publication of 'Parallel Distributed Process (PDP) Model' written by David Rumerhart, James McClelland James McClelland, along with Geoffrey Hinton, and 'Adaptive Control of thought (ACT) model' which was published in 1993 by John Anderson in the year 1993.

Memory development in the early years:

The important findings of William James in 1890 depended on the idea that the brain operates using dichotomous memories, both systems.They are primary memory and the secondary memory. The primary memory is information is stored for a short period as well as in consciousness stage.In secondary memory information is remains for an indefinite time and, upon request the brain is able to find the data.

Studies on primary memory, short-term memory, conducted by Joseph Jacobs in 1887 further demonstrated the capacity for the brain retain approximately 7 digits when tested by random numbers. He further established the possibility of having better memory ability if the numbers given are used for recalling in large groups or read aloud. In another series of tests carried out by George Miller in 1956, it was discovered that the brains can recall digits or letter as well as words with seven days on average, according to Joseph Jacobs in his findings and with a high probability of variances between 5 and 9.

What is the reason we lose information?

The opinions differ on what causes us to forget information.Until 1950, when John Brown, Margaret Peterson and Lloyd came up with a brand new theory regarding the reasons for not remembering, the most common view was that the conflict of information from the target with the latest information was the reason why we are becoming oblivious. The findings are part of the research carried out by Pilzecker, George Elias Muller along with Alfons around 1900. They were called'retroactive interference.'

The primary finding was that memory lasting for a long time is not associated to the process of learning however, it takes time to process the knowledge and in the process of consolidation there is a chance to forget what happened. According to new research, we are able to forget things because of the rapid decomposition of our memory trace and referring to it in terms of psychology as the neural substrate of the capacity to retain.'

How many memory systems do we have?

It was among the subjects that was hotly debated in the 1960s. How many memory systems are there and if it's two or one.Eminent researchers, such as Arthur Melton, always contented that there were no distinct memory component for short-term and long-term memory. Melton argued that the two are simply two components of the one system. Melton proposed a theory to prove his findings.However the new psychology has a convincing argument with the idea of having two distinct memory systems for the brain. The two systems are the short-term (STM) and short-term (LTM).

The year 1968 was the time that Richard Atkinson and Richard Shiffrini created the Multi-store model which was an accurate hypothesis of memory.It includes both short and long-term memory models, and then later an update that added'sensory' memory. The sensory memory functions as the short buffer zone prior to the information gets into shorter-term memory.Before the information enters long-term memory, it will be stored within the memory of short term that acts as an interim store device.The process of understanding and learning occur in short-term memory and is considered to be the 'cognitive task of memory according to the contemporary psychology terms.

In order to support the idea of short-term and long-term memories that is more real when compared to the two-memory theory, it is supported by a variety of aspects of memory, such as the capacity, the duration of limits, the speed at which memory is retained as well as the time it takes to obtain information, and information encoded, etc.

Systems and techniques for memory in the early days of memory technology

The development of memory techniques goes back to the Renaissance period, and was practiced by earlier Egyptians as well as the Pythagoreans.Even even though there isn't any conclusive evidence for the practice of techniques for memory in the

Egyptians as well as the Pythagoreans are believed to have employed the simplest types of techniques for memory. The Pythagoras was an ancient Greek mathematician and philosopher and the founder of Pythagoreanism.

The reference to the 'art of memory' are evident in the earliest works of Rhetorica ad Herennium, Deoratore, Institutio Oratoria and in numerous works of literature from the time period that dates from 400BC. The author of the first work is not known and the third and second are written composed by Cicero and Quintilian. It is fascinating to know that the well-known Greek philosopher Aristotle wrote about Art of Memory in his literary works, such as "On the Soul" and "On Memory and Reminiscence."

Ancient people came up with methods to master the art of remembering by linking place of origin instead of order of things or things that have happened.It is a method that advises people to focus on the location where events take place instead of recalling the specific event. This, in the future will aid in linking the place and the event, helping to recalling the memory.The traditional theory behind the Art of memory goes to Simonides of Ceos, famous Greek poet, who accidentally invented the idea of identifying deceased, whose body was found to be damaged beyond recognition shape, through recollecting the seat of the dignitaries who died.

The earliest Christian missionaries had the habit of employing this method of learning to remember Bible by studying the dialectical and rhetorical context which made it easier for people to retain Bible passages. The missionaries' helped people to learn the art of memory which allowed them to focus easily by reciting the Bible verses.

The theory of memory from the past focused on the selection of areas to translate that into mental images rather than recollecting events on the basis of that the order in which the area will help in remembering the order of things that will probably function as a wax writing-tablet technique.This method was employed by all the early Christian Missionaries to promote their faith and to instruct the Bible as well as other holy sermons to help their followers understand and recall the holy scripts.

The renowned Italian friar Giordano Bruno, also proposed an alternative form in the Art of memory. He explained the system of memory as arguing that "the mental faculties of the person who is practicing by presenting images that represent all the knowledge of the universe, in a magic sense, opens the way to access the world of intelligibility that goes beyond appearance and ultimately allow individuals to significantly influence the things happening in the real world." The 16th and 17th centuries were the time when the science of memory developed further with new scientific techniques and mathematical interpretations.

The efficiency in the field of memorizing came up against opposition from a variety of famous scholars, like Puritans, Erasmus and many.They were of the view that the effectiveness of memory was directly linked to the quality of memory, with a well-organized disposition to ensure a quick and accurate retrieval of memory.

The fundamentals of memorization are the following categories: spatial and visual perception and order, as well as restricted sets association, affect and repetition.

Chapter 3: Benefit of Meditation -- Simple and proven methods for positive Changes in the Brain

Everyone has, in the past known about meditation as a method of enhancing brain activity. In the preceding chapters, the use of advanced brain imaging as well as serotonin synthesizing enhances its efficacy. In this chapter, we'll want to start with the obvious changes in the gray matter of the brain in response to meditation, and then move on to simple practices of meditation that you can begin today to experience positive brain effects that improve mental health, mood as well as psychological and behavioral outcomes.

A study recently released in Psychological Science revealed that even shorter meditation sessions produced significant changes in cortical activity. Indeed, a researcher in University of Wisconsin University of Wisconsin discovered that the group of people who were enrolled in short meditation sessions that were not more than 25 minutes experienced similar changes in cortical activity that those who participated in the full-length sessions.

This study suggests that short meditation sessions can result in massive positive changes in emotional activity within the brain.In fact meditation is only one of the tried and tested practices that dramatically alters cognitive function , and over time, users can experience a tremendous positive growth of the new neural pathways. A study on memory found that meditation can increase the amount of grey matter in the hippocampus, which is that is responsible for memory and learning and memory, and decreases the amount of grey matter in the amygdala, which is the area that is that is responsible for brain's alarm systems. The evidence of these changes in the brain can be seen in the evidence that supports the brain's ability to change due to meditation.

Here are some simple to learn meditation techniques that have been used and proved to create positive changes in the brain specifically in terms of emotional stability as well as learning and memory management. The first strategy I present is simple and is best used as in preparation for the more advanced techniques of meditation.

A simple Breath Awareness meditation

Choose a peaceful and relaxing place where you won't be distracted

Maintain your spine straight in a chair, with your feet on the ground

Then, you can begin to observe your breathing and increase your curiosity regarding where it travels into your body and the way it departs

Be sure to not alter your breathing technique Simply breathe in a normal way

It is quite common that your mind is occupied particularly in the early stages when you start to practice meditation. Make sure you gently return your mind to your breathing and without being harsh or judgmental or in any other way.

Concentrate on your breathing for 15 to 20 minutes.

Although this practice of meditation is not difficult but its efficacy is established. But, it's only the tip of an glacier when it comes to meditation. Next step is to integrate mindfulness into your meditation practice.

After a few sessions of slow breathing , and then gentle redirection your thoughts (as they drift occasionally) your next task is the habit of rewiring your brain.As you begin to recognize the moment when your mind wanders contemplating, establish a regular mental habit to pay attention to every random thought for what it occurs, acknowledge it for a second and then accept the pattern and then slowly return your attention to your breathing.

When you repeat this exercise several times, you can include some systematic counting while you return to your breathing, such as counting 1 for inhale and 2 for the exhale . Then repeat. You can also use mental phrases to describe the action like "I exhale", "I exhale".As you make your counts or and add words to the action, this improves your ability to concentrate on the present moment of awareness . It also increases the accuracy and strength of neural signals associated with concentration.

It is essential to remember that you should take in thoughts and not become angry or irritable when this occurs.Simply accept that our minds are composed of thoughts, and we are able to think about them, acknowledge all of them, and yet have the ability to manage them and focus our attention on what we would like to see.

To add a layer of meditation, you might be able to sit and observe one object for at most 5 minutes, taking in its form, color and even its feel. It is also important to think about the object in terms of the reason it exists it's purpose, as well as what your life would be like without it. The object you choose doesn't require any specific features. You can just as easily choose a random object every day, whether outdoors in the home, inside or in the office.

The goal of the whole thing is to stimulate your brain's neurons in a manner which is distinct from your routine and is focused on your current state of awareness.Meditation is most likely to be the most efficient and fastest method to achieve brain change.As mentioned earlier there is evidence that brain chemistry that includes serotonin generation and a rise in axonal and myelin levels and enlargement in the more sophisticated areas associated with emotions indicate that there is value in repeated meditation. The best part about this all is it does not matter whether you meditate for hours or just for five minutes. You change your brain regardless. It's fascinating to realize that you aren't stuck with a non-growing, stagnant and aging brain? The area of Neuroplasticity is intriguing and complicated, yet benefiting from brain plasticity shouldn't be difficult in any way.

Chapter 4: Focus on What's Most Important

We all desire to be successful or lead the life we take pleasure in. In order to achieve this it is essential to not to get distracted by achieving things that aren't important. It is essential to grasp the secret to maximize every aspect within our life. If we're honest about ourselves, this isn't as easy to do than say. It's more theoretical than in practice.

This capacity to squeez every drop of our energy to be able to fully enjoy all aspects of life isn't found. Are we chasing after money? It's not because we don't ever seem to have enough. Does it come from climbing up the corporate ladder? Not really, since even if we reach the top of the ladder it is not enough to be content with our achievements. There is a chance that you will lose friendships with your family members in the process. So how do we optimize all aspects of our lives without losing anything? What are the actions we can take to take advantage of life to it's glory?

These are the issues this brief and easy ebook book aims to solve. It's an in-depth look at making the decision to pay attention to the most important things. This is a statement on the thing that you must to give all of your attention on in order to be successful in every aspect that you live in.

If you make the decision to increase the impact of this single area, you will witness the world change dramatically within your life. Five years later and be glad you chose to beginning this journey.

Are you curious about the basics? Okay, let's jump into it now, and then.

Power of Your Head Power of Your Head

In the animal kingdom, humans are considered to be the most distinct out of all the animals. Lions might have more strength than us Eagles can fly faster than us and sharks are able to swim better than we however, somehow we have ruled across the entire planet.

We've developed vehicles that shield us from the lion's attack as well as planes that fly higher than eagles and built ships that dominate the ocean. We have become the leading power on the Earth and even to a level that we know that we are the only ones capable of protecting our planet.

It begs the question what gave us the power to use this power? If it's not power, speed or body frame What gives us this unique advantage? If you've ever thought in your brain, "It's our brain" and you're right, then you're right.

The thing that's separated us from all other species of earth is our brains. That is, you were screaming within your brain, "It's what is in my head!"

It is due to our brains that we've created complex technology that has transformed the way we live our life exponentially over the last 100 years. It is due to our brains that have been able to break through the standard death barrier and begin to reap huge amounts of wealth that people decades ago could have only imagined. We have witnessed important medical breakthroughs as our brains have been devoted to tackling the most serious diseases that we face today.

In the present, as our developed brain has granted us the ability to live and rule on Earth What do you believe could to further enhance this advantage in our life? Yes, it's your brain.

Simply said you brain could be the single most important thing you can ever put your money into and be focused on throughout your life. The focus you place on your brain will enhance every aspect of your life, to a level where you can be able to see the fruits of your labor and know how the brain in your brain can produce enormous results.

It's so crucial that it will allow you to reach unrivalled levels in your personal, professional physical, spiritual and interpersonal life. It is able to make the most ideal life that anyone would want, just by mastering all its intricate aspects. From controlling thoughts to developing memory strategies one can enjoy an endless amount of accomplishment (which could be considered a personal word instead of a broad declaration that functions as a "one size is not enough for everyone") within their lives and in their lives because they devoted all of their focus on believing that what's inside their minds is of highest significance.

The Journey Ahead

As we continue to work towards finding out the ways your brain can be used to improve every aspect of your life and the small steps you can take to attain these outcomes, there's one thing that you need to take care of and that's something crucial. If you don't accomplish that one step, you'll not be able harness all the information described here and watch your life alter. The one thing being demanded of you commit to the process to make your brain the top thing that you own.

The reason why this phrase can be described as a"journey" is due to a variety of reasons. It is first as it sounds: it's a journey which basically means that you won't finish it today, tomorrow or one month from now. It's a day-in, out commitment that requires commitment in order to see it come be completed. If you're not dedicated to it then you'll make excuses. If you're committed, everything will be fine or stop you from doing it - not even yourself.

The second reason is that travel isn't straightforward. Some are more enjoyable than others. Some areas are more rewarding and others are just must tackle to ensure moving on to the next stage. The potential of your brain may not always be a rainbow and a rose. There will be actions that bore you (like supplementing your diet daily) and some things are fun (like being able to remember fifty people's names).

It is also an experience as your knowledge grows as you progress along the road to personal excellence. There might be things we discuss that are timeless and can be useful for years in the future, but certain things could be outdated in five years' time. You must be flexible to flexible and hungry to maintain your growth and knowledge to ensure that you are always better than you were yesterday.

If you've decided to make the commitment (and this is about making yourself a firm commitment that is not an easy one) If you've made the decision to commit, then you're prepared for the next step. You're prepared to begin realizing how increasing the power of your brain will enhance your life. Now is the time to concentrate on the things that matter most to you.

From here on we will look at the process of you can make your brain your primary concentration will improve these areas:

Professional

Emotional/Relational
Spiritual
Physical

Let the journey begin.

Chapter 5: Understanding Brain Plasticity And How It Really Works

The process of brain plasticity is often called cortical remapping or neuroplasticity. It is the capacity that the brain has to transformation and to adjust to the various experiences an individual experiences. Before the 1960s, researchers considered that the brain could undergo changes only in the early years of infanthood and early childhood. However, as we have seen in the first chapter in this compilation it is evident that adults are able to develop their cognitive and mental abilities by utilizing the brain's plasticity.

Brain Plasticity History

The man who made the suggestion Was William James, a psychologist who was the first person to suggest that the brain's structure undergoes modifications, contrary to widely held belief.This theory was proposed at the beginning of the 1890s. He stated that the nerves and the brain tissue according to his theories are likely to have the ability to reach an adequate plasticity. For a long time this idea was rejected and even against by some "experts" within the discipline.

In the 1920s in the 1920s, It in the 1920s, it was Karl Lashley who was first to offer evidence based on research and science that indeed, there were changes take place in the brain and are visible in Rhesus monkeys. In the following decades the discovery, researchers began looking into the instances of adult (in older ages) who had suffered strokes and recovered their functions. This is a further example of how malleable the brain can be.

These are just a few of the studies that demonstrate ways in which the brain could be conditioned to change and reconfigure its brain to adapt to the environmental stimuli.

How does the idea of brain plasticity actually work?

In all, the human brain is made up of nearly 100 million nerve cells. The conventional belief is that as soon as a baby is born neurogenesis (or the development of neurons) ceases. This is a myth that has been debunked since there are studies that show that our brains are capable of creating new neurons and making new nerve connections.

Here is the most important facts you should learn about brain plasticity or neuroplasticity:

The degree of plasticity can change with the age. It is a process that can occur over the course of your life. There are certain kinds of changes that are prevalent at certain stages of life.

The brain's plasticity process involves a myriad of processes. It's continuous and begins at the beginning and continues until the end of our lives. Apart from neuronal cells, the process also includes the glial cells as well as vascular cells.

The process of brain plasticity could be a result of any one of these caused by damage to the brain or as a result of learning, memory development and experience.

Environmental influences in processing brain development. Genetics can also play a role in determining the process.

The initial years of life for humans are essential because the growth rate of brain cells is fast. From the moment of birth, neurons in the cerebral cortex are believed to contain around 2,500 synapses. After 3 years the birth, the synapses could increase sixfold (up up to 15,000 synapses).

Adults on average, have between 7,500-8,000 synapses. Why is there a decline? Neurologists say that it is caused by synaptic pruning. As we get older connective tissue get stronger, but there are some which are cut off. Connections that are used frequently tend to be more powerful. The connections that aren't being used eventually discarded.

Are there two different types that are brain-related plasticity?

Based upon research, there are two kinds of brain plasticity, namely functional as well as structural. Functional plasticity is the capacity for the brain change its functions from areas of the brain which are damaged to areas within the brain that aren't damaged. In contrast structural plasticity is the ability to create structural changes through experiences and learning.

Chapter 6: Understanding Evolutionary Medicine

Evolutionary medicine is a fascinating area of science fiction for a long time. It was a topic that captivated the minds of many dreamers, too. Recent years have seen that evolutionary medicine is beginning to demonstrate some promise. It could be said it is on the path to making an enormous contribution to the modern society. In the near future the hopes and dreams of evolutionary medicine could very possibly be a reality in the in the near future.

One of the main focuses of modern medicine is the power for technology to be used as a method to improve the health of our bodies. Technology can be utilized to improve the natural functions of the body or to take these abilities to new levels.

Technology, for instance, can be utilized to improve cognitive performance. It is possible to help people become more intelligent by increasing their concentration in order to improve memory retention.

In the present, technology is being utilized to help damaged body parts or replace diseases or parts that are untreatable or not treatable. Examples include the robotic legs and arms which respond to brain's signals, just like the real human arms and legs. It's a massive leap to making use of prosthetics made of plastic that move or have any function other than use up the space that is left over by body parts amputated

The field of evolution also offers creative concepts. It suggests that technology can be utilized to offer specific, well-defined enhancements in a short time. For instance, upgrades can help slower body processes, like healing. For instance the body can treat a minor superficial injury in around four weeks. New cells are created to replace damaged cells, and also to heal the wound. Following the healing process the area appears as like it was never damaged in any way.

This is a lengthy process. The effects are also limited. The more complex and severe injuries can only be partly cured through the body's healing process.

Through the use of technology, the inherent ability is enhanced to heal more severe injuries in an even shorter time. Imagine the Xmen character Wolverine and his remarkable self-healing capabilities to a certain extent. This may not be an instantaneous healing process but it is much faster than current rates or even a few weeks.

The concept of evolutionary medicine to be a method to enhance your body's performance was popularized through Amal Graafstra. The ideas he proposed are based upon the basic notion that the body could be modified to perform greater than it is able to do. He suggested that technology could be implanted in lieu of hands to turn knobs in order to open doors, or to input a security keys to open security-locked doors. He decided to implant an DIY RFID (RFID) inside his arm. This allowed him to open the security locks on devices and activate connected lights and smart devices with one swipe of his RFID-implanted arm.

What Graafstra performed was just an illustrative example of the kind of evolutionary medical treatment could be. There are other less extreme instances that many people are enjoying today.

Quantified Self

The concept of the quantified self a notion that is widely believed to represent a pathway to evolutionary medical. It is a concept that is similar to biohacking as it suggests that the human body can be enhanced when paired with technology. This isn't similar to making human Cyborgs.

Quantified self is currently used by a lot of people in the present. There are numerous wearable technology which can measure the amount of steps taken as well as calories burned, muscles that are used in specific exercises as well as the rate of pulse blood sugar levels as well as blood pressure. There are running shoes that determine the kind of terrain you are that you are running on via GPS and the length of runs. This data is then recorded in applications which can be used to track the progress. All of these fall in the realm of the self that is quantified.

The information collected by these devices could be used to make changes in activity, diet or lifestyle, sleeping habits and goals for health. They can also be used by health professionals to aid in determining the best treatment to the person's needs.

Self-evaluation is an effective way to motivate one to become more involved in taking health of their body. It can also be a great assessment tool for the exercise regimen as well as training sessions and treatment techniques.

This method helps people feel more empowered and active. The people now feel that they are more in control of their health.

Combining the ideas of biohacking and quantified self, there's the possibility of significantly increasing the efficiency of the body. These two elements play key parts to the development of evolution in medical research.

Information is getting more accessible to a larger percentage of the population through wearable technology. The people of today have more control over and direct involvement in many bodily tasks. The time is coming when this control will extend beyond just making changes to the diet, exercise and treatments. These will be used to assist the body to function to the fullest extent possible and to become a more effective human being of the future.

Chapter 7: Neuroplasticity And Brain Repair

How Neuroplasticity is activated in the event of damaged or impaired Brain Cells
Injuries or diseases can harm or destroy brain cells. In this situation neuroplasticity kicks in to aid the life systems of the person affected by constructing new neural pathways and redirecting crucial brain functions to brain cells that are not affected - overriding damaged neural connections during the process. The aim is to limit the injury to the affected region and avoid any further problems by dispersing functions of the brain to normal

brain cells that are located elsewhere in the brain.

In tests conducted on rodents, it was demonstrated that normal brain cells that were located in the surrounding area of the damaged region were able to perform the functions as the injured cells instantly after they underwent some changes to their form and function. Additional findings from these tests show that the exact same thing occurs in the human brain following an injury.

Neuroplasticity and Stroke

Stroke is the 4th leading reason for death across the United States. The patients who survive will experience the most drastic decline in their quality of life as a result of permanent impairment. It is a serious threat to the brain that can seriously affect your mental awareness and capacity to learn, think, communicate or walk and also solve issues.

The primary cause of a stroke is the disruption in the flow of cerebral blood. Without blood flow, glucose and oxygen will not get to the brain cells, thus starving the cells to death as a result. But, functional recovery may happen naturally even when blood flow is not restored. In reaction to brain injury, neurons in the vicinity of damaged cells begin creating neural pathways that connect with other neurons in order to create neural circuits that will replace the functions of damaged cells. Additionally there are also'mirror neurons' located on the opposite part of the brain (opposite to the area where the brain damage occurs) that can assume some of the functions of the damaged cells.

Neuroplasticity is slamming into action to perform brain repair in the crucial time following the occurrence of the stroke, the time when there is an increase in the amount of brain plasticity. There are lots of people who don't know about neuroplasticity, and they are more likely to give up on any hope of recovery once initial rehabilitation therapy is unsuccessful. However, for those who understand there is a way to train the healthy regions of brains to replace the functions that were lost with the hope of stroke victims achieving more than a functional but full recovery is not just optimistic, but is also more than likely. In actual fact, there are numerous successful cases of full recovery of stroke victims , which proves the significance of neuroplasticity in the process of brain repair.

One such tale is that from The Dr. Jill Bolte Taylor, one of the brain scientists from Harvard who had stroke at 37 years old, that left her completely disabled. She was unable to walk or talk, read or write. Also, she lost the ability to recall the memories of the past. In other words she lost all her motor and cognitive capabilities.

Jill began her career as a brain scientist due to her brother who was diagnosed with schizophrenia which is a brain disorder in which patients experience hallucinations and delusions. She was determined to discover the differences between the brain circuitry of her brother and hers , and why her brother was experiencing hallucinations and delusions whereas she did not. She was unaware that she would experience the firsthand experience of having her brain's functions affected each time through an accident. She had no idea she would be able to recover from the stroke , and then share the remarkable story of her recovery to all of us. Her story seems to be an unheard of, God-given research opportunity to learn about post-stroke recovery as seen through the eyes an expert in brain surgery who lost her mind because of a brain injury caused by stroke.

Jill's road to recovery took her eight years. Even though she couldn't speak or walk, she was during her entire ordeal, aware of what was happening in her environment. The left side of her brain was injured. As a scientist in the field of brain, she was well-versed in neuroplasticity, and she knew precisely what was happening in the brain. She recognized that it was the left-brain that had been affected. Her brain would be redirecting functions to the damaged brain onto the brain of the right. The best part is that she was aware of exactly what she needed to do: she would be the designer in her own mind.

When Jill determined to take the first step towards recovery, she knew she needed to be focused on the process. She began working on her movements, mindful of the fact that she had to learn everything from scratch by taking one step at a. She began by rocking in the bed, every single day, to raise herself up until she could finally be in a position to sit straight. She was putting herself to the test every day by taking baby steps, slowly over the course of eight years, until she completely recovered her mobility abilities and cognitive abilities.

As Jill Stroke patients need to be aware of how neuroplasticity functions to help them to accept the challenges of recovery. The road ahead for people who have had strokes will be difficult because it will test their already limited physical and mental capacities. It is only when they push their bodies to the limit that be able to stimulate the brain to work faster - and create the necessary functional adjustments to the healthy cells so they can take on the functions of the damaged ones.

The difficulties that stroke victims have to confront include learning to re-learn the lost skills of speech, motor and language skills. It's a difficult task for someone who has totally lost his motor and cognitive abilities as described by Dr. Jill Taylor together many others have demonstrated that it can be accomplished. Every step of the process of recovery is similar to working the brain to stimulate neurons, and is no different than those of a young child who is learning how to walk for the first time.

Chapter 8: Limits of Self Hypnosis

Self-hypnosis should only be employed as a tool, not to get away from reality. A lot of things is, as the old saying goes, is harmful. Self-hypnosis isn't always being useful and is destructive.

The primary drawback of self-hypnosis comes from it being the case that every methods involved in achieving the state of hypnosis are performed in the exact same way by the same individual. In order to master self-hypnosis it takes a considerable amount of practice and time is needed to master the skill and be able to execute it consistently. The procedure of achieving an hypnotic state that is self-initiated is fairly easy, but it is a bit of effort necessary when you need to utilize this method for reaching the objective. Many people try repeatedly and even if they don't notice any changes, they will quit. This is a mistake and also a drawback when it comes to self-hypnosis. The people who learn to use self-hypnosis must be patient and persistent since the effects of self-hypnosis are cumulative and will require repeated sessions to see the effects.

Many people try self-hypnosis and then, if they don't notice any significant changes or effects will then decide to stop self-hypnosis. The main reasons for the low success rate of self-hypnosis include:

A person may not have the ability to comprehend the root of their issues

Research has proven that your capability to assist yourself will only be as effective as the ability of you to be open and honest about the root of the issue is to be tackled. The process of identifying these issues is an issue if we don't know what they're all about. A clear and accurate evaluation or judgement is needed on the issues that need to be dealt with, but the majority of people lack the viewpoint and objective. Many people will find excuses and strategies for denying or denying the reality of what's going on even when this denial doesn't serve their long-term interests in the world. You may be denial about your issues and defense mechanisms or strategies for denial make it difficult for you to discern the causes and the root cause. Because you are unable to resolve what you don't understand it is unlikely that you'll be able to resolve your issues through self-hypnosis. You could end up creating additional issues instead.An person may not have the understanding of how to solve your problems.

Another issue that a person could face is working out the best way to resolve the issues that they face. This is especially true for those who are honest and precise regarding the nature of their difficulties. For success with self-hypnosis, one must have a thorough information. The information is about the root of the problem and what can be addressed. The issue is that it requires access to resources as well as the determination to read and research the sources before you are able to solve the issue. There is no way to be born with the skills to know the best way to tackle problems and not all are prepared or ready to do the effort.

A person may not have motivation to continue using self-hypnosis

This is another issue that a person faces when doing self-hypnosis. Many individuals may be aware of the requirements they must meet while performing self-hypnosis, but they fail to stick to the program. Finding and keeping the desire to stick to self-hypnosis is one of the biggest issues.

Other limitations of self-hypnosis include:

Obsessed or failing to make the most of self-hypnosis: People are likely to fall into the routine of doing a hypnosis routine every day until the brain is unable to take an opportunity to connect and take in the lessons learned in the hypnotic state. Self-hypnosis shouldn't be used for more than 5 days one week.

Self-hypnosis isn't at a place to resolve certain issues that a person may be facing. Problems that are complex and can affect an individual at the highest level and create extreme personal stress should be handled by professionals. Issues like depression trauma, anxiety, and destructive behaviors should be addressed. the person seeks out professional help that will include counseling and individualized therapy.

There is debate over which method is more effective professionally-managed hypnosis and self-hypnosis. The efficacy of any form of hypnosis is different depending on how an individual reacts to the sessions. One complaint that self-hypnosis can receives is that it doesn't necessarily result in a change in behavior.

Self-hypnosis is not a factor that affects the body's structure in ways that go beyond biological. This means that it isn't an accurate assumption that self-hypnosis will aid in gaining inches in size, get rid of cancer or reduce weight. Self-hypnosis is a method of facilitating changes put in the body by the person who is hypnotized however, the changes only affect physical processes. For instance, self hypnosis is not a cure for cancer, but it can aid in reducing the negative effects of treatments like chemotherapy. Self-hypnosis is sure to aid in feeling more balanced and calm.

Chapter 9: The Exploration of Conceptual Spaces

Applied spaces are structured styles of thought. They usually originate from one's own lifestyle or a friend gatherings, but can also be acquired from various social groups. Whatever the situation, they're in existence, but they weren't created by a single person. They encompass methods of writing poems or expositions and styles of figure music, or painting as well as hypotheses from science or chemistry; patterns of fashion or movement, new cooking techniques, and delicious traditional meats and veggies simply any trained viewpoint that is recognized by (and appreciated by) an individual social group.

In a particular space, various possibilities are possible and a few could have been considered. Certain spaces, clearly possess more exuberant possibilities than the others. Crosses and noughts are an incredibly limited style of playing that every move that could be possible has been played out numerous times. However, this does not apply to Chess, in which the number of moves that could be made even if they are small, is colossally large. In addition, if sub-regions in science have been diminished (each possible particle of that type being identified) The space of possible limericks, or poems, hasn't ever been.

Whatever the dimensions of the space, someone who thinks up a new idea in this reasoning style is creative and imaginative in the second more exploratory sense. If the thought that is conceived is astonishing by itself, and also in the case of an unimaginable general kind, that is the ideal scenario. Additionally, in the unlikely possibility that it leads to others (still within the same space) that were previously unassailable, that's even more impressive. Exploratory creativity is crucial due to how it could allow someone to consider results that they had not previously considered. It is possible to consider the limits and what possibilities, this approach to thinking can bring.

You can see the contrast between this with the crashing into the country by using the Ordnance Survey map that you advise on a regular basis. It is possible to stick to the motorways, or just look at the red lines on your map. Whatever the case suppose that, for no reason (a police call or an emergency from nature) You drive away to a smaller street. When you arrived the road, you had no knowledge of it. Of course in the event that you open the guide, you'll find it positioned on the inside. Perhaps you contemplate 'what's at the corner or around the corner?' And then you drive it around to see. It could be that you drive to the town of your dreams or a home for a committee and find yourself on a circular drive or return to the motorway you escaped in any event. Each of these scenarios could have been conceivable (and they're all talked about in the book). Yet, you've never encountered them before - and probably likely wouldn't have in the unlikely event that you weren't in an exploration mood.

In exploration-based creativity, the concept of "open country" is a way of thinking. Instead of exploring an organized geoological area it is a more structured applied space that is which is defined by a particular way of painting or even a particular area of imagined science.

Every professional craftsman or researcher performs this type of work. In fact, even the most common road-based craftsmen from Leicester Square produce new representations or personifications frequently. They're examining their surroundings but not necessarily in a bold manner. Every now and then they might realize that their style of drawing allows them to achieve things (pass on the layout of the head or the traces of a smile) that is superior to what they've done before. They can add another item to their arsenal, however in the real sense, it's an act that fits their style of drawing The potential was always present.

Transforming the space

What road experts might also do is to understand the limitations of their design. They also have an open door that drivers on the street don't. With or without the years while ignoring earthquakes and floods, the nation's streets are in good order. You can't alter them. The Ordnance Survey Map is trustworthy because of its privilege and in light of how it's correct. (Have you considered purchasing another guidebook in the last few years?) But the maps we have in our minds, and supported with our social networks could be altered - and it's our creative thinking that transforms them.

Some changes are very small, and also relatively thin. (Ask yourself: What's an actual difference?) The boundaries within the mental guide or of a specific portion that is minimally moved, slightly altered or tinily altered. Examine the situation in topographical space: imagine that each of the townspeople has suddenly has added a roof to their home. This could ruin the charm of the town, but it will not alter the basic elements that comprise the book. It's likely that the tiny'representation of town (assuming that it's the same sort of guide) must be revised.

The road craftsman or Picasso or Picasso, in a similar position , has a chance. At a basic level, the road craftsman (or like the usual or she) might be able to create the psycho-consistent resemblance, including roof enhancements, or constructing a different street (another method, resulting in different possibilities) or even re-directing the motorway.

Redirecting the motorway (in real life, or it appears in the mind) is the most challenging of all. The shocks that it could cause can be so amazing that the driver could be compelled to lose direction. It is possible that he will think the mysteriously transported to a different region or even another country. Maybe he remembers a puzzling incident from his last trip in which he was required to complete something, but his traveler snidely stated"In England motorways operate the same way. They just aren't able to allow this. Do you have to do it? Intense! It's inconceivable.'

A certain method of reasoning, although certainly not a street-level framework, may make certain ideas unimaginable or, more precisely impossible. The distinction, as mentioned earlier is that reasoning styles are able to be altered - just several times with the flick of an eye.

A person who has mastered the art of writing an original limerick is unlikely to see versifying pentameters falling from their pen. However, on the chance that you're required to compose another type of limerick or a non-limerick, in any means or other, and anchored in that well-known style or style, then maybe a clear and concise the refrain can be used to do. The most significant examples of creativity are when someone is thinking about something that, for the spaces that are calculated within their heads, could not think of before. As far as anybody is aware of, the outlandish idea could be a result of the creator alters the prior style of thinking here and there. It has to be altered or completely altered considering that there are some considerations possible that (inside the space that is not transformed) were a mystery. But, how will this occur?

Mind maps for machines

To understand the ways that transformative creativity or exploration occurs, it is important to understand the theoretical space and what kinds of mental processes could be used to explore and change them.

The reasoning styles are viewed by musicologists, abstract pundits and historians of workmanship scientific and design. They are also admired by everyone. Yet, their natural gratitude and even the long-lasting grant, could not be able to reveal their design. (A specialist in compositional history such as this one, has said about Frank Lloyd Wright's Prairie Houses that their 'rule of solidarity' is 'difficult'.)

This is the main reason that computers play a role. Reasonable spaces, and the methods to study and transform them, are portrayed through ideas derived from human-made conscious (AI).

Man-made intelligence theories allow us to conduct brain science in a different manner and allow us to create (and test) theories about the structure and the processes related to thinking. For instance structures of toneal agreements, or the'sentence structure' from Prairie Houses, can be clearly communicated, and specific ways of analyzing the space are available to give an attempt. Methods of exploringand changing deeply organized spaces are studied.

Naturally, there's always the issue of whether the suggested methods and structures are actually implemented in the human head. Additionally, this issue isn't always simple to answer. However, the idea is that computational thinking provides a means of formulating logical theories about the complexities of human brain.

Computers are creative

What is the relationship between machines and creativity? Are computers able to be creative? But, on contrary do they at all do anything but show all the signs of being inventive?

A lot of people believe that no computer is creative, no matter what its design resembled. Whatever the case, regardless of whether it beat the average road-creature or researcher but it isn't thought of as innovative. It might have theories as revolutionary like Einstein's, or music that is as awe-inspiringly revered as McCartney's "Yesterday" or Beethoven's Ninth however that for these people the music would not be considered innovative. There are a variety of arguments typically used on the other side of that. It's for instance that is it the engineer's creative genius that's churning away in this instance and rather than the machines. The machine isn't aware of its needs, desires or desires which means it isn't able to recognize or make a judgment about the work it's performing. Show-stoppers are a result of human emotion or an exchange between people and machines, which means that they do not have the ability to tally.

Perhaps you have recognized in some case one of the motives that computer programs are not able to be creative? Well, I'll agree with you. Give us the chance to recognize that as the ultimate objective of this exchange computer don't always have the ability to be creative. The most important thing to remember is that it doesn't mean that there's something more essential to mention.

All of the complaints listed acknowledge, for dispute that the computer's imaginative appearance is like that of people regardless of how low or high. What I want to focus on is whether the data prove that computers can create thoughts that appear to be, in all appearances, to be imaginative.

Computer-related combinations

If you think about it, consider combinatorial creativity first. In one sense, it isn't difficult to show using computers. It is no more difficult than picking two ideas (two data structures) and placing them in close proximity. It is feasible with a little nuance making use of connections (connectionist). In a nutshell: computers is able to create novel combinations until the time of death.

In any event, could they be interesting? We discovered that consolidating thoughts creatively isn't as appealing as moving marbles around in a group. Marbles must be joined on the basis that there exists a comprehensible yet unnoticed interaction between them that we value because it's intriguing, enlightening creative, intelligent everywhere. (Think of resting and sewing again.) We also saw that combinatable creativity usually requires a abundant supply of information of a variety of kinds and the ability to form connections of a variety of types. (Here take a look at legislators and newts again.) We don't just make joints, we also evaluate them. For instance, we may detect that a joke may be "in bad taste". That is to say, truly the connections the joker suggests are real (so it's a real joke). There are many other connections that connect the thought with sadness, remorse or even disaster. The person who made the joke should have noticed them and should have avoided the temptation of bringing them back to us.

To make a casual joke about combining that doesn't hesitate to look at its sophistication, is going to require, in the first place the existence of a database that is the same amount of information as ours, and, in addition, methods for connecting (and connect evaluation) nearly identical in terms of the way we do it. In a fundamental sense this is not a stretch. In all likelihood brains and minds don't perform this feat through the magic of enchantment. But, whatever be that, don't put your hopes on the line!

The most successful example of computer-driven combinational creativity thus far is a program known as JAPE it makes clever jokes that are common to all eight year olds. However, composing a singular joke is usually more difficult. Consider, for instance the information Jane Austen needed to know to come up with the first line in Pride and Prejudice: 'It is generally accepted that a single man with a good fortune must have an heir.' (And what exactly is it funny?)

Artificial explorers and self-transforming robots

Why shouldn't we talk about the power of exploration? Some projects today are able to explore the space in appropriate ways.

One example is AARON which is a drawing program. AARON produces thousands of line drawings that are drawn in the style of a particular style, which is satisfying to be awed by being suddenly observed by astonished guests and then displayed in exhibitions around the globe and even Tate. Tate.

Another one is David Cope's Emmy The music is composed by David Cope with a variety of styles that are reminiscent of human writers like Bach Vivaldi, Mozart . . . and Stravinsky. Some projects incorporate structural elements that design Palladian manors, or Prairie Houses, and other projects that are suited to breaking down research information and identifying more effective ways to communicate logical laws

Some AI-related projects can change their theoretical world by altering their own theories so that fascinating ideas emerge. Certain of these thoughts were then well-known to humans, but they were not specifically incorporated into the program. But, as it happens other programs are new to the market. "Transformative" programs, for instance are able to roll out random changes to their current guidelines, with the intention that new kinds of structure result. Every cycle, the best structures are picked and used to create the next generation of people to follow.

Two models that are advancing color-coordinated images (some of which, like the AARON's are featured in museums around the globe). In each case, the selection of the most 'fit for each age group is determined by an individual who selects the most aesthetically pleasing examples. In simple terms they are clever illustrations of scenarios, where humans and computer work together in the creation of images that would be otherwise impossible. Computer-

81

generated images often trigger the third, and most powerful kind of shock that is, as if an object that was thrown multiple times were at once to display the most bizarre design. In these instances there is no relationship between the tiny girl image and the parent. It gives an impression that it is an extreme alteration of the other or perhaps something completely different.

Anyone who has sat on the couch in front of the television frequently in the past few years, or has visited historic centers of modern-day craftsmanship you will be aware that many new and realistic images were created without the help of any other AI-related projects like this. The problem isn't making the changes, it's usually easy. The problem is to communicate our esthetic preferences clearly enough to enable the program to perform assessments at all ages. The "common determination" is made by a particular person (for example the guest on display).

In spaces that are more directed in better-directed spaces, be that as it could, the worth criteria can be articulated in a way that is clear enough for the transformative program to use them naturally. A first model. Researchers are now using these methods to boost their own creative abilities. Biochemical labs in universities as well as pharmaceutical organizations are employing innovative projects to create new particles that can be used in vital research and prescription. In fact, even the 'brains or groups of robots will soon be able to advance rather than being designed.

Chapter 10: A Few Of the Most Common Mental Models

The great thing about the cognitive

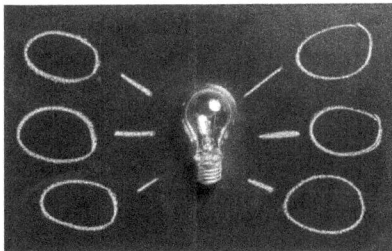

models is that there are many of them that you're in a position to use. This lets you think and behave in a variety of different ways, and it can assist you when it's time to make a big decision. In this regard this chapter will examine the top ten mental models however, there are at minimum 80 of them that are applicable to our current world. The top ten mental models we will concentrate upon in the next chapter comprise:

The Map Is Not the Territory

The reason we are going to use in this model is the way that we choose to perceive the world doesn't necessarily reflect the reality. The worldview we've got will base itself on personal mental model. Maps are just going to be the mental model we employ. Territorial boundaries will change with time, and everything around us may also change.

From a larger perspective, the idea that the map isn't the actual territory. It can help us avoid some of the logical errors that happen when we misinterpret labels or semantics with things which are actually real. The other errors that are similar to this include the misplaced concreteness and the idea of reification. Each of us will have our own mental map which helps us see the world. But the world is complexand it's impossible for humans to comprehend everything that is happening. Therefore, our assumptions and beliefs, as well as our assumptions and conclusions will not prove to be the best indicators always helping us understand the fullness of the world.

When we are ready to examine our interpersonal and communication relationships It is probable that we'll try to project our own mental map on others, or believe that they ought to be able to discern the mental maps we have created. But , it is important to recognize that the people who interact with have their respective mental maps and they'd like us to follow their maps instead of our own. This is where the majority of confusion, miscommunication and, sometimes, extreme conflict are likely to occur.

It is indeed possible for two individuals being in the exact spot and possibly even experience the same scenario or situation and then come away with a completely different experience. Based on these different experiences, we'll be able to discover that there are various views and perspectives that are involved. If this is the model you're going with, be aware that you shouldn't try to dictate your beliefs to others. Instead, strive to understand yourself and also accept the worldviews of other people.

There are a variety of ways you can use these mental models to your everyday life. This includes:

Making decisions

Management of relationships

Leadership

It is the Circle of Competence

There isn't a person who is able to have all the knowledge available. There will always be gaps in our abilities and information that we have. It is crucial to recognize the things we aren't aware of. It's not a problem to not be able to know everything, as it's simply not feasible. Staying focused on what we know and observing how they can help us move forward in our lives is much more beneficial.

By completing the circle of competences through the circle of competencies, you will be able open your mind to further learning. You'll be able stay clear of common misconceptions and errors throughout the process. It is possible to get rid of the ego-based ignorance and increase understanding the ability you possess.

This will help you a lot. It will help you determine your strengths as well as your weaknesses. It can guide at the way you must take to break free from the trap of failure and enable you to meet the right people to enable you to gain knowledge from them and increase your skills. A few of the various tools that you could use to expand this circle include:

Advancement and career development

Making decisions

The First Principles Thinking

It will be more about detaching the fundamental information and ideas from the assumptions you can make. When you use the principle of first thought it will allow you to break down a problem into its elements and the root causes in the present. It is much easier to tackle these issues in the most efficient way, instead of rushing around in hopes that you make the right choices on the way.

You can figure certain pathogens that trigger the symptoms of the disease. In this way, you can provide some relief to the illness and not just relief from the symptoms you are experiencing. By focusing on the elements that make up your body You will discover the elements to create something completely new. Some of the possibilities you'll encounter in this regard are:

Making decisions

Problem-solving

Engineering

Chemistry

Medicine

The pursuit of Knowledge That is Liquid

Solid knowledge will consist of pellets that will be gathered into silos. As an example, you can have a biology silo maths silo, physics silo Silos, and so on. the knowledge that is solid is unlikely to be fluid or ever moving and rarely flows.

The most brilliant free thinkers will to transcend the rigid knowledge taught in schools and discover the liquid knowledge that is uncondensed not refined, and flowing freely. The kind of thinking you are able to get will come from experience based on personal experiences your personal discoveries, and also from your own research. This lets you have an enjoyable time as you explore your own discovery of knowledge. This will make the process more enjoyable and enjoyable in the process.

Think Explore

Thought experiments are likely to be a tool of imagination, which are employed to study the nature of the objects that surround us. They will be vital whenever you are looking to discover new territories, particularly when you're trying to explore uncharted areas. The territory could be completely unknown and undiscovered to you or it could be a mystery to other people as well. This type of exercise will enable one to break the impossible, consider the possible consequences and then compare these results with the ones previously known ones to aid them in making certain informed decisions.

It is likely that differently from other tests you could conduct the thought experiment is likely be conducted solely within the mind, even being able to show it physically to show that it is true. This kind of mental model will come be called an experiment in the mind rather than.

Galileo is one of the scientists who participated in this experiment in order to develop some of the principles of science which are believed as valid to this day. Albert Einstein also used this method. The main problem with this type conceptual model of mind is the fact that without the ability to verify it through empirical evidence this is something is difficult to establish as being real or not. Therefore, there are philosophers who see it as mental models of the physical world rather than. A few of the uses of this model include:

It will help you investigate the design of your idea.

Simulation of scenarios and synthesis.

Exploration of the scientific method

Second-Order Thinking

The first concern we might be faced with concerns whether there's an First Order? Sure it is! Before we examine the Second Order of thinking, it is necessary to give an introduction of it is that the First Order is all about and then contrast the two.

If we're working with thinking in the First Order thinking, people will make decisions that are quick and hasty and dependent on what they discern on the surface or on the surface. Due to this rapid decision-making process, the person will not be able to dive deeper than they ought to to comprehend why things happen in the way they do. They react rapidly, based on initial impressions, not paying attention to the circumstances as well as whether or not they ought to respond with this way or not.

We then have the Second Order Thinking. In this type of thinking, the person will take their decision-making and thinking to a higher level. They'll be studying the basic principles that drive this phenomenon to determine the different elements that contribute to this.

People who use the Second order of thinking, instead of jumping into the decision or going to the conclusion too fast and making a decision too quickly, could take a decision that is contrary to the what they thought their First Order thinking would have performed. Let's look at an example of this. If there's an explosive that occurs, the First Order thinkers are going to seek to flee as they think the cause of the explosion is the explosion of a bomb, and they would like to escape the danger as fast as they can.

But then there are the Second Order thinkers. Even though they may want to follow their instincts and take flight, they will be more likely to pause and think about what it could be that caused the explosion, figure out if they are close to the explosion, and then figure out what they could do about it. Maybe they find out that it was just a big tire that burst by them and there was no reason to run off and be scared of it.

So, in some manners of thinking, the First Order thinkers are going to reach to the already existing mental image that is in the mind of this kind of thinker. The actual occurrence that shows up is going to just be the trigger for that action, but not the cause of the action.

Another good example of First Order to Second Order thinking is in the sphere of investment. For example, if Company A declares that there is a profit warning, most First Order thinkers are going to anticipate that the price of the share is about to fall. Because of this, they are going to rush to get rid of the shares as quickly as possible. This causes the shares to happen, but this is because the traders jump in too quickly, not because the value of the shares actually went down.

On the other hand, we can see that a Second Order thinker is going to have done the process of a fundamental analysis on the profit warning to figure out what is going to cause that profit warning. This could easily be something small, like a new investment decision that resulted in less profit, but a bigger asset base. This means that if you hold onto the shares, there may be a temporary dip thanks to the First Order thinkers, but overall, your value from the shares are going to heat back up.

There are a lot of different times when you will be able to use the idea of First Order vs. Second Order mental model to help you make decisions. Some of the best applications of this mental model are going to include:

Decision making of any kind

In a fundamental analysis

Investment decisions

Emergency response

Occam's Razor

This is a model that is going to posit that the simple explanations are the ones that are more likely to be true, rather than going for the explanations that are more complex. So, if you are using this mental model, you will find that it works the best if you can pick out a solution that has fewer assumptions in it.

What this means is that when someone makes a decision, they need to be able to minimize the assumptions as much as possible, with the help of experimentation, study, and research before they implement a new decision concept that they want. In case there is not a lot of leeway in the amount of time that is available, then the concept that has the fewest assumptions is the one that is considered the most ideal for implementing.

The reason for this is that when you have more assumptions present, the risk of having some decision errors is going to be higher. Some of the applications of this mental model is going to include:

Personal development

Career choices

Management

Leadership

Decision making

Inversion

The next mental model that we are going to take a look at is inversion. Inversion is the idea that you will think backward. With this one, you are going to create some likely scenarios after the action or decisions and then you need to seek out how to address all of the scenarios before you decide on which course to take, or before you decide to execute it. This means that you need to be able to approach the problem from the opposite of the natural starting point.

Let's take a look at an example of this. You may be considering a separation or a divorce from your spouse. Before you jump into this and go ahead with some of the divorce proceedings, by inversion, you would stimulate some of the potential scenarios that would happen with this. It could include a strained relationship with your in-laws, loss of your home, increased costs of childcare, loss of your partner, property division and more. If possible, you can then start to mitigate some of the adverse effects of these scenarios before deciding for or against the divorce.

To make this one work a bit better, you have to make sure that you attack your decisions by going backward. This helps you to really plan things out, imagine that things are already done, and consider what decision is actually going to give you the results that you are looking for.

Some of the different applications for the inversion mental model will include the following:

Career choice

Leadership

Decision making

Personal development

Family planning

Probabilistic Thinking

When you work with probabilistic thinking, you are going to use a variety of probability tools, including statistical tools, to help them approximate the likelihood that a certain event is going to occur. There are two major technologies that already use this including machine learning and artificial intelligence. Some of the different applications of using probabilistic thinking as a mental model will include:

Strategic planning

Actuarial science

Computer sciences, especially when we look at machine learning and artificial intelligence

Decision making

Investment

Hanlon's Razor

The best look at what the Hanlon mental model is all about is "never attribute malice to that which can be simply explained by stupidity". The gist of this is that you should never assume that something bad is happening because of the wicked intents of others on the situation. Sometimes it is just incompetence or stupidity on the part of the actor, rather than some malice on their part. Stupidity, in this case, can be from the other person, or from you. It is possible that your own stupidity is causing problems because you made the wrong assumption, but then it could be the stupidity of the other person as well.

Due to the egocentric view that most of us have of things, which, in our subconscious minds, assumes that everything in the world revolves around us, we end up assuming a prominent role in the story of everyone else, even though this isn't true. This means that when we are around someone who seems a bit annoyed, we assume that it has to do with us and that we have made them made. When another person is rude to us, it is because they are angry at us or just being mean to us. When we see that someone doesn't want to congratulate us, we assume that they are feeling jealous of us.

As part of the stupidity that comes with us, we are going to perceive some negative responses as malice against us, without being able to consider that it is often due to factors that have nothing to do with us. Hanlon's Razor model is going to be helpful because it can avoid paranoia, anxiety, and stress. It will eventually save us from taking a bad situation and making it worse.

When we use this mental model, we have to understand that to be human is to err, and that there are times when people make mistakes, and even we are going to make some mistakes on occasion. This means that we need to find out if there are other explanations for what has occurred, rather than assuming that there is some malice that comes with this. This is why with Hanlon's razor, it is always best to assume the best intentions or some good faith before we try to prove otherwise.

Some of the applications that we are going to see with the Hanlon's razor will include:

Relationship management

Decision making

Diplomacy

Conflict resolution

Crisis management

As you can see, there are a lot of different mental models out there that will help you to make decisions, based on the way that you see the world and the point of view that you are looking for along the way as well. Each of these can be effective and ill help you to see some of the results that you want with making decisions that are going to be based on sound judgment, rather than on our emotions or something else that can be subjective. You can determine which of these mental models, as well as some of the others we will talk about in this guidebook that you would like to use to help you make some good decisions and to ensure you can make the best decisions for yourself.

Chapter 11: Brain Plasticity And Localization

As we've discussed, brain plasticity (also known ascortical plasticity or neuroplasticity) is the ability of the brain to reorganize itself, forming new information processing connections and new functions for those cells. This happens:

*During infancy and childhood and into young adulthood as the young brain organizes itself.

*Through adulthood, whenever we form new memories or learn something new, or develop a new skill.

*In response to any brain damage or brain disease or congenital disorder, such as blindness, to compensate for lost functions or maximize remaining functions.

Recent evidence demonstrates that the brain is capable of remarkable widespread adaptation throughout life...much more than had previously been thought.

One remarkable type of brain plasticity occurs when parts of the brain that normally serve one cognitive function are taken over by other parts of the brain to serve other, completely different functions.

A general principle of brain function is what is called localization. Different perceptual and cognitive functions are performed by different parts of the brain. Damage to one part of the brain results in a highly specific and selective deficit, while leaving remaining cognitive functions intact. The following example is representative of brain plasticity to compensate for a loss.

Blindness From Birth

Blind individuals have to make some major adjustments in order to cope with and flourish in a world that is designed for the sighted. Blind individuals develop heightened abilities in the use of their remaining senses in order to compensate for the loss of sight. Their superior skills in tasks involving touch and hearing has been documented in laboratory tests.

The rear most lobe of the cerebral hemisphere is called the occipital lobe (see diagram). If this lobe is injured in sighted individuals. That person becomes blind. If a person is blind from birth and they learn to read Braille, a brain scan reveals that person's occipital lobe is being used for the sense of touch as the Braille is being read. One modality (touch) is substituting for another modality (vision), this kind of plasticity is called "cross modal".

In other research studies, it was found that the occipital lobe of blind individuals is being used for speech processing, a function that is normally performed in the temporal and frontal lobes (see diagram).

Examples of Reshaping the Brain

In one study, after just five days of blindfolding a normal sighted individual, the occipital lobe (see diagram) showed signs of processing touch and auditory information functions normally processed by the parietal and temporal lobes (see diagram). This is a rapid, temporary arrangement of brain structure and function, designed to adapt to new demands. The occipital lobe returns to normal functioning once the blindfold is removed.

Brain plasticity as a result of skill acquisition and extensive learning in specialist areas is the norm. Cortical territory shifts over time in response to the knowledge and skills we acquire is now expected.

Hydrocephalus

The brain is literally suspended in a fluid called cerebrospinal fluid. This fluid bathes the interior and exterior of the brain and the entire central nervous system (brain and spinal cord). Without cerebrospinal fluid the brain would collapse under its own weight. Hydrocephalus is a condition in which there is an abnormal build-up of cerebrospinal fluid. Without medical intervention, hydrocephalia can lead to brain damage and even death.

In hydrocephalia, fluid accumulates in the four pockets of the brain called ventricles. If the fluid build-up is not relieved in these ventricles, brain swelling occurs and the neural tissue is pressed up against the skull.

British neurologist John Lorber has documented over 600 scans of people with hydrocephalia and has categorized them into four groups:

*Those with nearly normal brains, little cerebrospinal fluid.

*Those with 50-70% of the cranium filled with cerebrospinal fluid.

*Those with 70-90% of the cranium filled with cerebrospinal fluid.

*Those with 95% of the cranium filled with cerebrospinal fluid...the most severe group.

The last group comprised 10% of the total brain scans. 50% of the last group was severely retarded. The other 50% had IQs greater than 100 (An IQ of 100 is considered average...certainly not retarded). One young man in this category of virtually no brain had an IQ of 125 and got first class honor degrees in mathematics! Brains are normally around 1.5kgs. But these cases prove that 50-100 gram brains may perform at a normal and even superior level.

Almost all that neuroscientists know about brain anatomy and function is now questioned because of these types of findings.

Neuroscientists point out that these findings explain another part of the puzzle that illustrates the extreme versatility and plasticity of the brain.

Brain Plasticity & Nature vs. Nurture

Up until around the 1970s it was widely accepted that throughout adulthood our nervous system was fixed, however, a new theory of brain plasticity, also called neuroplasticity has become the current accepted theory of how our brain ages.

This enlarged idea is the concept that the brain is able to reorganize neural pathways based on new experiences.

Basically, we continually acquire new knowledge and skills throughout our lives. In order for us to learn a new skill or fact our brain must undergo a functional change. When the brain changes to learn new things, that is brain plasticity.

Foot Print in the Snow

A great example of how neuroplasticity works is to imagine making a footprint in the snow. In order for your footprint to appear in the snow, a change must occur in the snow.

Plasticity plays a role in learning and memory. Research over the last two decades has uncovered two types of modifications that occur in the brain during learning:

*First there are changes in the structure of the neurons, primarily in area where synapses occur.

*Second, there is an increase in the number of synapses between neurons.

Nature vs. Nurture

It is interesting to note that genetics (nature) is not the single most significant factor that influences brain development. The environment that an individual occupies shapes the brain. Also, the experiences (nurture) of a person within that environment molds the brain.

The last few decades has seen a dramatic shift in our view of how much the brain is capable of changing.

Chapter 12: Behind The Curtain – How Neuroplasticity Happens

Neuroplasticity involves a lot of processes in the brain. It alters connections between neurons – neural synapses and pathways, and involves changes to neurons, vascular cells, and glial cells.

Neuroplasticity happens thanks to a process called synaptic pruning. This is your brain deleting neural connections that are no longer useful or necessary. The connections that are necessary, in turn, grow stronger.

You may be wondering how your brain decides which connections to prune out. This depends both on your life experiences, and how recently neural connections have been used. When your neurons are underused, they get weak from underutilization and die off through a process called apoptosis. In other words, neuroplasticity and synaptic pruning are your brain's way of fine tuning itself for efficiency.

Neuroplasticity can be brought upon by physical trauma. The body may heal itself from injury, but the brain adapts. Many times, physical injury would otherwise result in loss of function in the body. Yet, when someone does lose function after suffering bodily injury, the plasticity of the brain can come to the rescue!

It occurs in two ways:

During normal brain development when the immature brain begins to process sensory information – like when you were a baby and learned to walk. Or through adulthood as an adaptive mechanism to compensate for lost function maxing out remaining functions after brain injury.

The Mind

Everything you just read above describes the physical elements of the brain. The mind, however, is altogether a different business. As much as we use both terms interchangeably, they do not mean the same thing in any way. The brain, as you saw, is a tangible organ that you can touch and feel. The mind, however, is intangible, and is more of a mental construct, than a physical object.

The mind uses memory and extrapolation (which can be referred to as imagination) to develop a kind of pseudo-reality within our head. The mind uses algorithms that are based on occurrences in the real world and then extrapolates them to understand and predict an outcome.

What we retain in our brain and the method in which we retain it is not as simple as we may think it is. For instance, what we see is not what we remember, rather, what we remember is an impression of what we see. That's how it is for most people. For the rare few who remember things as they see it, they are referred to as those who possess a photographic memory.

The same goes for what we smell, and what we hear. It is all subject to interpretation before it is stored. This is true no matter how strongly you believe that you remember things the exact way they occur. Two people can witness the same event but because the brain interprets information before it stores it, they will have different ideas of what happened. Their recollections may be similar, but they will not be the same. Problems can arise when one person thinks what they remember is right, therefore, they think the other person must be wrong. When in actuality, they are both right. They just interpreted and stored the same event differently.

So, we have the photographic memory and the normal processed memory. Photographic memory can be learned, believe it or not, and it can be practiced. The key is that you need not possess a photographic memory, which is on one side of the spectrum, or have a processed memory, which is on the other side of the spectrum. The trick is to have a healthy balance of both. This doesn't mean that you sometimes chose to remember somethings in one way and other things in another way. What it is, in reality, is that you learn to remember all things in raw and processed ways, but you do so, to different degrees, in two different phases of your brain. More on the phases of your brain in the next section.

Phases of the Brain

If you are wondering why we are still talking about the brain when we are supposed to be talking about the mind, well it's because the frequency, or the phases it creates, are very much a part of the mind. It's like radio frequencies. The frequency created by the brain is like that of a radio station creating a frequency so that it can place its programming on top of it. In the brain's case, thoughts and emotions ride on top of the frequency that the brain creates.

In this section, we are not referring to the stages of brain development. The brain is not divided into compartments based on physical separation like the hard drive of a computer. Instead, it is based on different frequencies. The conscious and awakened state, the state that you are in now as you read this, is at a frequency that is relatively lower than your subconscious state. Your subconscious state works at a much faster rate and can hold more.

We are unconsciously operating under the belief that we write our memories and that it no longer matters if we are awake or not. That is untrue. One of the reasons our brains takes up such vast quantities of energy is because our brain is constantly serving it cells with the energy it needs to maintain cognitive functions. If we were to stop the blood flow to the brain for just three minutes or deprive it of oxygen for the same amount of time, what we will find is that the brain is the first to shut down.

The brain is no more static and passive than the heart that beats and has been beating since before the brain formed in the womb, and which will continue beating till the last breath. The brain, on the other hand, will continue to live for approximately three minutes after the heart stops.

In that way, it's like the RAM in your computer. It is volatile memory - keeping what is stored only while power is supplied to it. The moment power is disengaged, everything is lost.

The brain operates on various frequencies that can be observed when it is attached to an electroencephalograph (EEG). The neurons and cells that are in the brain are involved with the passing of electrical energy and with an EEG that is the source of the image that is then produced. If a specific area of the brain is stimulated, then that part has more electrical activity and that is the area that lights up on the EEG.

What we consider as thoughts and what we consider as feelings are both just different wavelengths of electricity that runs through the brain. Your subconscious happens at a much higher frequency, while your conscious occurs between a little over 0 Hz to about 500 Hz. That's about all you can detect. Above that frequency, detection by your consciousness is fairly minimal, but you can feel it. If it goes higher than that, you would not be able to feel it.

For instance, all the things that are going on in your subconscious are happening at a much higher frequency. Different parts of the brain run at differing frequencies. To understand this better we should look at the concept of brain waves. Stay with me. This is amazing stuff, and once you get a better understanding about what is going on in that brain of yours, then you will be able to master it. You will be in the driver's seat, and you'll be able to steer your vehicle in the way you choose.

Brain Waves

Depending on how deep you want to take it, there are numerous wave categories. But for the purpose of this book we will look at just six. These brainwaves are at times referred to as the speed of the brain and it is easy to fall into that trap. What brainwaves are, instead, are the speed at which the electrical impulses pass in repetition through one or through a group of neurons.

Frequencies are measured in hertz. Hertz normally is the representation in seconds. So, for instance, 60 cycles per second, or the repetition of sixty impulses in the span of one second, is said to be 60 Hertz.

The brain technically can't do 0 Hz. And it can't do negative Hertz, either. The slowest that has been recorded is at below 0.5 Hertz and even then, it's a difficult process as detection becomes immensely problematic. The top end hasn't been quite determined yet, although there is a theoretical limit at about 100Hz. All the measurement that happens extracranially is typically detecting the impulses that are happening in the cerebral cortex.

To visualize, imagine this: Take one neuron, from its cell body, across its axon and down to the axon terminals as a wire connected to a switch. Imagine the myelin sheet to be the rubber insulation on that copper wire and imagine the lightbulb at the other end of the wire as the dendrites.

Imagine if you were to turn that switch on and off once every second. An electrical impulse will flow through the wire and reach the bulb, illuminating it. If you increased the amount of times you flipped that switch on and off, the bulb would flash on at a faster rate. The faster rate corresponds to a higher frequency.

In the event, that there is no impulse at all, that is considered death.

Neuroscientists and psychologists have agreed on several bands of frequency. Ranging between just below 0.5Hz and 50Hz with rare but possible frequencies that have been thought to reach 200 Hz for those with intense meditation ability and those experiencing states of enlightenment. We have chosen, as mentioned earlier, six classifications. In some medical circles, there are more, and in some there are less.

Infra Low Waves

Occurs below 0.5 Hz (but greater than zero). This is rarely studied because of the lack of technology in detecting such low frequencies. However, it is theorized to be a state in which the mind is at total rest.

Delta Waves

These are waves that occur between 0.5 and 3Hz. Unlike Infra Low, these are easily visualized in EEG tests and relate to periods of deep meditation. If you invoke these waves prior to learning and study, you will find that memory is easier. But do note, that it does not mean that learning in other frequencies are futile. On the contrary, learning is not just based on the frequency of the mind, it is based on the frequency of the input. If you match input frequency to the frequency of the cerebral cortex, then you have a better absorption rate than you do when they are not in sync.

Theta Waves

These waves are measured between 3 and 8Hz. This is what you get in deep sleep and in some forms of deep meditation. Deeper meditation will put you in the Delta range. Once you are at this level (approaching from a faster cycle down to this), you are leaving the external world of bodily sensations and the environment around you and are able to focus completely internally.

Alpha Waves

Here the waves are measured between 8 and 12Hz. When you practice mindfulness, this is the state you will be in. It is a superior state to be creative and to allow ideas to flow. It is the ultimate definition of the here and now, and the thoughts that come to you in this state are highly imaginative.

Beta Waves

These waves are between 12 and 38Hz. At this frequency, the brain consumes high quantities of energy, requiring constant replenishment of nourishment. But nourishment alone is insufficient as the brain also gets tired when operated at this frequency for too long and requires rest or it is faced with the risk of damage. Any stresses on the brain, including running it at Beta, should be done incrementally and allow the brain to get used to the operating speed before sustaining that speed for too long. This is especially true for Beta and Gamma states.

Gamma Waves

Occurring between 38 and 42 Hz, these waves signify a state of heightened awareness. The brain is able to process input from various channels more efficiently and at a highly accurate state. The thing that conventional researchers find hard to reconcile is that this frequency is above the rate at which the neurons are thought to be able to fire. So, the question that traditional neuroscientists pose concerns the alternate source of wave energy that drives this Gamma state. Some also believe that there is a possibility for spiritual awakening and super consciousness at this frequency.

As a student of neuroplasticity, it is not important that you commit these frequencies to memory. They will come in handy but what you do need to understand is that the underlying functionality of the brain comes from the oscillations of electrical energy that pulses through the neurons.

The Gamma state is really the highest state in which frequencies can go up to levels beyond 200 if practiced meditation is undertaken. Contrary to popular belief, meditation is not the calming of the mind, that is mindfulness. Meditation is about the heightened focus of the mind. At the highest states of meditation, ESP and large quantity data processing can occur.

It is also observed in meditators who achieve these high rates of brainwaves that they can experience time dilation. Time dilation is the mind's ability to interpret time. Without turning this book into a high-level physics text, it is sufficing to say that it has already been proven that time is unique to each of us. There is no such thing as common time. What you see on your watch is not time, it is man's attempt to measure and quantify time, as well as commoditized time for the purpose of scheduling.

When you increase your brain waves out of the gamma range, what you will find is the brain's ability to dilate time, therefore, it will be like fitting an entire hour, day, year, or decade into mere seconds.

All this would not be possible if the neurons, or a bunch of neurons did not exist. Because, as you have already seen, it is the neurons that act as conduits for these electrical impulses.

Chapter 13: Benefits of Neuroplasticity and Positive Thinking

The study of neuroplasticity is becoming so well-known in recent times, particularly among psychiatrists who are the most renowned. The concept of neuroplasticity in psychiatry has become a notion that's spreading fast. It has had a significant impact on different treatments for diseases such as schizophrenia, depression, addiction, anxiety, as well as other serious diseases that are managed by psychiatrists who are experts.

Positive thinking is a powerful tool. Have you ever heard the phrase mentioned? It's become a regular part of our everyday life that it's almost irrelevant. It's a fact that being positive is positive. Particularly when we're feeling happy.

What happens the times when things get tough? What happens when you're stressed to the point that you're unable to think straight? Are you able to cope with those days when you're caught off guard by numerous events that overwhelm you.

We've all met people who are extremely positive when they are in a downer. Between us and you I feel like smacking them occasionally. The whimsical, "life is beautiful" attitude when things are crashing actually got out of my system.

However, I've learned that these people had a knowledge I did not.

The secret isn't any longer a secret. It's an exciting, revolutionary scientific. Positive thinking actually alters your brain. Not in a hippy, woo-woo sort of way. It alters your brain's structure in a physical way.

Neuroplasticity is the science behind it. It implies that our thoughts can actually alter your brain's structure as well as function. The concept of neuroplasticity was first proposed around 1890, in the work of William James, and it was widely dismissed by scientists who general considered that the brain was tightly mapped, with specific brain regions controlling specific functions. The consensus was that if one part was injured or died it would be altered or even lost completely. Now, it's beginning to appear that they were all wrong.

Neuroplasticity is now widely recognized as researchers begin to show it is capable of morphing and changing.

The brain has the ability to alter its own structure. This is even for people with serious neurological disorders. Patients suffering from issues like cerebral palsy, strokes and mental illnesses can alter the structure of their brains by performing regular physical and mental exercises. The research is proving that this can be life-changing.

What is this got to do with positive thinking?

This is because repetitive positive thoughts and regular positive activities could rewire your brain. It helps strengthen specific areas of the brain that are able to trigger positive feelings.

With his ground-breaking book The Brain It changes Itself The Brain That Changes Itself: Personal Stories of personal Triumph in The Frontiers of Brain Science, Norman Doidge M.D. declares that the brain has the ability to change its wiring and/or create new neural pathways when we do the effort. The same is true for exercise: it needs repetition and effort to help reinforce learning.

Here are some steps you can adopt to transform your brain's perception during tough times.

Fearing the risk of failing

We all fear taking on something new, and we aren't afraid to make mistakes. But the truth is that we are able to do almost anything if you take action, stop negative thoughts, and alter our views regarding our abilities.

Steps to take:

Stop and think about all reasons why you're not able to accomplish something even if you're not feeling confident or confident. When thoughts of negative thoughts creep in then redirect your mind to creating a positive image of your capabilities instead. Start taking small steps every day towards achieving your goals or achieving the desired change.

Over-thinking/Worrying:

Have you felt trapped by the midst of a constant over-thinking process or in an agitated state anxiety or stress that can last for weeks or even days? It drains your energy, disrupts your sleep, and stifles your mood and outlook on life. Being obsessed with your problems just increases the worry-related function within your brain.

Steps to take:

If you're caught trapped in the cycle of worrying or compulsive thinking, try the three R's - reframing, renaming, and redirect. When the worry starts, mentally shout "Stop!" Rename the problem by reminding yourself worry isn't an actual thing. Make it a knee-jerk reaction, not an actuality. Reframe your thinking by choosing to focus on things that are positive, or diverting, regardless of whether or not you feel stressed. Instruct your mind to think of other things. Change your focus. Find something stimulating and stimulating, exciting or stimulating. The true gold lies by following these steps over and over again each time you feel concerned or anxious to break the cycle and reset your brain.

Mood Disorders/Phobias

Sometimes, we may feel blue or unwell, but it's merely a temporary fog that passes and clears after a couple of days. Certain mood disorders, such as anxiety or depression that turn into phobias can be debilitating and persistent. Therapists and psychologists have employed therapies based on neuroplasticity in order to discover the underlying cognitive causes of these conditions and get the patient's life back in order.

Steps to take:

A serious disorder of the mood or phobia needs the assistance from a certified counselor. CBT, also known as cognitive behavior therapy (CBT) is one kind of treatment that assists people discover and alter destructive patterns of thought that can have a negative impact on their behavior and emotions. If you are suffering with depression or anxiety that is severe You need a professional to assist you in identifying the root of your thoughts and teach you how to alter these thoughts. Talk to them about CBT.

Scientists are looking into neuroplasticity to tackle a range of cognitive issues and diseases, such as:

The loss of sensesvision, balance, and hearing

Reading problems and learning disorders

Prolonged processing of the auditory nerve

Hypersensitivity and autism

Memory loss and the aging brain

Love and sexual relations

Recovery from brain injury and stroke

Cerebral palsy

Chronic pain

Obsessive compulsive disorder

Traumas from the psychological

Depression and anxiety

Cognitive problems after brain surgery

Neuroplasticity and anxiety treatment

The theory of Neuroplasticity is the idea that our brains continue evolving throughout our lifetime period. Another study has proven that brain cells in people who are suffering from anxiety suffer each day, which leads the brain to undergo negative plasticity. Researchers have attempted to correlate these two findings to study the ways that neuroplasticity could help with these disorders. The practice of neuroplasticity and the formation of regular positive thoughts along with neural connections has restored and assisted many in recovering from brain cell damage due to anxiety.

Neuroplasticity and depression

A lot of people who have experienced the trauma of a loss experience sadness, isolation and have a feeling of despair. They enter a state of severe depression at which they are unable to communicate with anyone, and they live in their own world. They could be silent or speak in a non-sensical manner. The causes behind this type of depression can be numerous. It could be because of any accident or loss of loved ones or a breakup or sudden loss in business , or any other stressful event. The primary effect of depressive moods is the damage to brain cells. The damage can be reversed and positive feelings can be instilled to our brains via practicing neuroplasticity. Experiments and studies have demonstrated excellent results when treating depression patients through neuroplastic therapy.

Chapter 14: What happens in The Brain when Habits are formed?

There are many small things we do every day without considering them. Showering dry or using our phones when we go to work, and even brushing our teeth are just a few examples of this. These routines are part of our daily routines and our brains create habits around them to complete these tasks without thinking about it a lot. What's happening inside our brains as we learn about a new routine?

What are some things is something you carry out on a regular every day and you are able to complete all of it without being thinking? This could be closing the door to your home before leaving. You could be on the way to work. Have you been in the position of getting to the destination you were going to, but aren't sure how you got there. destination. This is an excellent illustration of the autopilot state that brains can create when you begin to establish routines.

Habits are actually the basis for a lot of the activities take place in our daily lives. It happens so often that, even when we're looking to change our habits it is difficult to achieve because the behavior is deeply embedded in us. Habits that are good and bad are part of the autopilot brain mode and it's difficult to break it without a lot of effort.

Although we tend to think of the habit of doing things as a negative thing however, they actually serve as beneficial tools. Once we are in routine, and get into a habit of doing something for a certain amount of often that we master it with little or any effort. This has been recognized for many years. For instance, Aristotle reportedly believed that excellence wasn't really a thing however, it was more of a way of life.

We've spent a amount of time to study patterns and how they may be created and shaped, but what we're going to look at now is how this process is likely to appear like in the brain. What do neural networks react or behave when learning something? And how will this alter when we apply repetition to make it an established habit which we don't even consider.

Researchers from MIT took to heart. They have recently completed a study that included a lot of findings were released in the publication Current Biology. Let's look at this study and see what it revealed about what happens inside the brain after habits begin to develop.

The neural signals are redirected to bookend.

We develop habits every day. It's easy and simple. Sometimes we don't realize that we're forming the brand new behavior until we reflect and discover that we have a variety of negative habits to address. It's amazing that the majority of tiny habits we establish throughout our lives are just a series of tiny movements which are all necessary to carry out the task. For instance, we might be driving into work, without ever thinking in the past, and is now an everyday habit however, it involves many other minor actions that are required in order to get to work. It could involve getting outside and unlocking the car, reclining in the car, altering the settings of the mirrors using the seatbelt, driving down the road, and taking off the vehicle when you arrive there. All of these steps are for getting us to work early in the morning.

This intricate set of movements which can lead to complete a particular routine and especially when it occurs without conscious thought is known as chunking. We know that this sort of movement exists, however there's still lots of questions as to how the chunks are formed and how they can be stabilized in the brain.

The latest study carried out in collaboration with MIT indicates that certain cells within the brain responsible for rearranging the segments that are linked to certain habits of behavior. In a different study, researchers from MIT discovered that the striatum area of the brain which was previously linked with decision-making and decision making, can also be a major factor when it comes to the development of the habit of a person.

The team took time to study mice. In this period they observed how the signals transferred between the neurons of the striatum. These patterns changed when mice were taught a different series of steps. This was observed when mice began to move in one direction, when they heard a sound signal given while they were moving through the maze. At first the mice were taught to turn in this manner. However, over time the practice began to develop into a habit.

At first, when mouse learning was taking place, neurons within their striatas released an endless stream of signals, according to tests conducted. However, over time, as the mice repeated the same things over and over and over again, the actions of the mice began to develop and eventually become more routine. As this happened the neurons that generated the distinct signals took place at the beginning

, and again after the completion of the exercise.

If this pattern of signaling begins to develop and if it has already begun to take root it means that the new habit has begun and breaking free from the habit could be very challenging. This is a great option if you're trying to create an entirely new habit that is healthy, however it could make it difficult for people who are trying to break the habits they have had already developed.

Brain patterns that are a sign of patterns in the brain that indicate

While they were enlightening, the team at MIT observed that their previous research didn't prove that the patterns of signaling observed in the brain were connected to the formation of habit. The signals could have been just a few motor commands, which were used to control the way mice moved around or through the maze.

They decided to do some of their research in order to prove their hypothesis that the patterns which were correlated with the chunking could be connected to the development of habit. MIT came up with a few ideas to use. In the second study they conducted they decided to train rats to press two levers in a series however, they'd need to perform it in a particular sequence.

To encourage these animals, researchers employ a technique called reward conditioning. If the animals press the levers in the correct sequence, and after they learned the significance of this the correct sequence, they would receive chocolate milk. If they didn't press those levers with the proper sequence, they won't get the milk.

To ensure that there were no variables and there weren't doubts regarding the results and to ensure that the team could later discern the patterns in brain activity associated with the development of habit patterns, and not any other reason, the researchers were able to teach the animals several different kinds of sequences.

As soon as the test began and the animals learned how to perform the correct sequence. Once they were able press their levers using the correct order they were taught to do, the group noticed that the bookending pattern was showing up in the striatum. The neurons will be able to emit signals at the beginning of the task , and again at after the task was completed. This would then be able to remove a chunk of the task and allow you to complete it in a more automatized method.

It is believed to demonstrate that there is an underlying pattern of bracketing that shows up and becomes apparent as you begin to form an habit. They develop to make it easier to categorize a specific kind of behavior, or a set of them within a set of routines, which the brain considers useful and ones that the brain will want to remember to be used later.

Another thing the researchers observed was a development of a second type of pattern, which is complementar, within a set of inhibitory brain cells which known as interneurons and can be found inside the striatum. It was discovered that these interneurons were activated in the course of the experiment when rats were in the middle of executing the sequence they were instructed to perform. These neurons may be present to stop the primary neurons from starting another sequence until the current one is completed.

This is an excellent thing in most cases. It allows the person, or animal to remain focused on the same thing and not get distracted during it. It is not a good idea to start your commute to work only to discover that you're about get out of the vehicle, or find yourself to the opposite direction on the route. Understanding how these interneurons perform is an excellent way to help researchers better discover how brain's circuits actually handle this type of activity so that we can develop routines.

Chapter 15: Non-conventional Methods to Reprogramme Your Mind To Change Your Mind

Your Belief System

Your beliefs about yourself and others will affect your success and happiness in the future. A majority of our beliefs come by the things we consume and absorb in our surroundings. The views and beliefs of our family and friends as well as our exposure to media can have a profound impact on our perception of ourselves and our position on the planet.

As a result, it's possible to say that our beliefs are born from our environment and the way in which we interpret our experiences growing up in the same environment. It tells me two things. If you're able alter the way you perceive your environment, then your views about yourself and the world will change as well. So, by changing your beliefs about the world can help you alter your thinking, which can ultimately bring about a more positive life.

The ability to change your mind to change from a restrictive nature to an empowering one, starts with a crucial choice.

You can quickly assess yourself on how you believe and feel about yourself. You'll know if your current beliefs are beneficial to you, or merely restricting you.

Consume Positive Material

Scott is committed to the notion of "how to make the most of the world?" and improving your productivity. Through holistic learning, he breaks into simpler concepts to make them more memorable while demonstrating the real pleasures of learning.

Recently completed a four-year MIT degree in just 12 months.

He is a master of learning in-depth. He also tackles the many issues that many struggle with, like finding purpose and meaning in our work.

Tiny Buddha

Tiny Buddha is a website that promotes simple wisdom to live complicated lives. It's not just about giving you the basics in terms of material that is positive and offers suggestions for applying it. The blog posts cover motivation, happiness, inspiration passion, love and opportunities, mindfulness and let go.

Chris Guillebeau

Chris Guillebeau is a man who has a passion for challenging authority. Never ever having an "real job" to this day, Chris is dedicated to living life on his terms and being paid to do the things he enjoys. His aim is to assist people to live a life that is unconventional and make their own decisions and transform the world according to his own style.

Make a Pinterest Account is a social media site that is built around images and the things you cherish in life.This is an excellent way to discover hidden phrases to boost your mood throughout the day. Every day, dedicate yourself to finding quotes and pictures that inspire you to be happy. The more you are exposed to positive images and positive people who make you feel happy, the more quickly your perspective will undergo a positive shift.

Read to read, read and read.

Consider this as treating it as a religion.I'm sure I'm not kidding.If you truly wish to reprogram your mind you should take the following.Figure out what beliefs are holding your back.

Develop the beliefs you'd like to be a powerful force within your mind's makeup using methods like affirmations.

Others who write about personal development like my own are always striving to bring harmony and joy in people's lives. across the globe. Instead of reading the boring status updates that people post in their accounts on Facebook and Twitter Why not check out the most popular 100?

personal development sites and regularly read them instead?

Additionally, instead of taking a look at the newspaper that lands on your door every

143

day. You can tune in to the positive news paper?

2. Create Your Own Beliefs , and then Monitor Your Environment

The people who help us through the toughest moments of our lives are truly friends. There's a distinct distinction between an acquaintance and true friend. The former is the one who is always there to assist you in times of need. A bad friendship group can just make you feel miserable.

Contrary to what many believe there is more benefit when you're on your own rather than in a group with negative people.

3. Be skeptical of everything and everything you are currently adamant about:

"People lead their lives by what they consider to be truthful and correct. They define reality in this way. What is it being "correct" and "true"? Simple concepts... They truth could be a figment of imagination. Are they just be living in their own universe that is guided by their opinions?" - Masashi Kishimoto The need to know what others believe is the primary obstacle to realizing their goals. I care about what others think, but I consider the opinions of people who I admire.

4. Keep a personal Positivity Journal

The only restriction is that you're only permitted to write positive thoughts in the journal. Writing in your personal positive journal is a wonderful method of boosting your confidence in your self. After six months, you can begin to believe in yourself again.

For the next several months, you'll be filled with an abundance of thoughts, motives thoughts, stories and concepts that will allow you to see the truth of it all. You are a much better person than you believe you are.

Chapter 16: Establish Good Habits

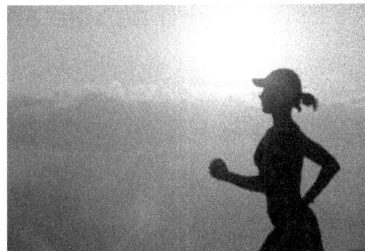

Concentrating to get rid negative habits isn't enough. We must incorporate positive habits into our lifestyle.

I hope that you've continued to focus on the interruption of thought for those unwanted positive or negative ideas. You've even thought of an idea to do something new or revisit your childhood child. It's time to think about the person you are and what you'd like to achieve in your life. There are a variety of ways you can take care of yourself frequently to prepare your body, mind, and your spirit to be the best version of you. Let's examine a few of them.

It is important to prioritize relationships

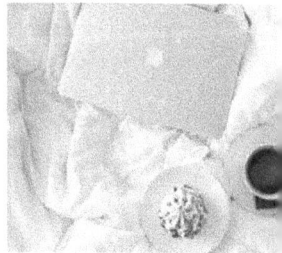

with people and not things.

In today's information-saturated society, it has become natural to pull out our phones whenever there is any amount of downtime. If you take a look at those who are waiting in line everywhere in the city, in the stores or waiting to get seated at restaurants, they are constantly sitting or standing with their heads downand with their phones in their hands. Why would they do that? Our phones can play games that are fun or chat with friends and read blog posts, or news stories, and keep up with our celebrity friends... But wait for a moment, did we not already talk about getting rid of the information overflow? That's right. It's time to focus on your interactions with others. Let's create a small task for you to take on this week.

If you are going to the supermarket or the bank or perhaps even when you go out with your family for dinner take your phone out of the car. What?! This is exactly the way I described it. Put your phone in the car. When you're in line-- which can be nerve-wracking at times, try making a nice gesture to the person who is behind or directly in front of you. I know...you may get some confusion, perhaps they're too caught up in their phones to even notice you or maybe it will be too long since they've heard real human interaction that they won't be able to even think of what to say. But I challenge you. Engage with someone on the line and then observe what transpires. Chances are you're going to have a positive encounter that'll stay in your mind for the remainder all day. People really enjoy talking with strangers in the store. Many people experience an enormous boost in their mood from even the tiniest interactions like this. However good it feels after receiving an email or a liking on your Facebook page, it's not likely to be the same as real-life interactions. Therefore, do yourself a good deed and try to make contact with people you don't

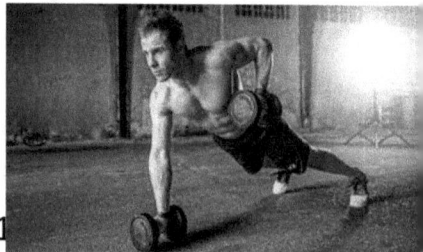

know every week, at least.

Let's focus on the relationships you have with your close friends, family members and/or family. Consider a person you consider to be a acquaintance that you haven't spoken for the past week or so. What's the reason? Perhaps it's because you've been overloaded with work? Are you juggling children? You've made it clear that other aspects of your life should take priority over your friendship with your friend. I'd like you to think about whether you've had too much on your plate to squeeze into a phone call lasting 15 minutes with your friend. Perhaps you're too exhausted from work, and you've not made it an effort. It's something I'd suggest you shift your mindset. Friendships and human relationships are among the most significant aspect of life and it's unwise to give up precious time with these people to watch Netflix and pizza every evening during the work week. It's true that work can be exhausting and you'd like to go home, relax and get away from the world. We've discussed this before, as well. Why would you want to waste your life in this way? If your work is so demanding that you're unable to focus on anything else, and you are so eager to escape it that it's impossible to work during the day, perhaps you should reevaluate your career options. However, I'll let you arrive at that conclusion within a matter of minutes. Your current task is to choose an appointment this week to get out and meet to one of your most loved people to have a chat, and perhaps dinner. If you're not looking to shell out on food, invite them to your house and arrange dinner together. Perhaps you'd like to head to their place because it is quieter...that's okay! No matter what you do, the most important factor is to set the intention of spending time with your friend this week. This is a great habit that you'll enjoy a lot from. More than the cup of Moose Tracks ice cream in the refrigerator!

Keep the journal going and track your progress. Journaling is fantastic method to keep your mind focused and track your improvement. It's important to have a written journal to refer whenever you're feeling like you require some encouragement. Make a point of writing a portion of your journal each daily. Write about your feelings and what you've been able to overcome over the past few months and your determination to persevere. This is also a good way to stay on track. Note down the things you've challenged yourself to complete this week, and note immediately after you've accomplished it. Continue to work, and eventually you'll have pages of work that you can take a look at when you're struggling or in need of some motivation. We all have these days, and it's fine! As I mentioned before it's a huge task. It's essential to not let your goals transform into chores or sources of stress, just like the ones that you've worked to eliminate! Be challenging, but be careful not to burden yourself too much. Don't try to tackle every advice in this chapter all at the same time! I've laid out a few alternatives in the hope that there are certain ones that stick out as something that could dramatically improve your life as well as your thinking processes. Keep in mind that no one can make a huge difference in their lives in a matter of minutes!

Be aware it doesn't need to be a mere collection of words. If you're like me , and you love motivational quotes or beautiful images, you can use your notebook or your journal to create a kind of scrapbook. You can include photos of cartoons, quotes and even tickets stubs, birthday cards and ticket slips that you could be tempted to throw away. These are a lot of fun to reflect on and you'll be grateful that you kept the items in the future.

Eat better
Be healthier, not "eat healthier." I've put this in the context that there's no better method to stall your progress than by

overloading you with an obstacle that requires you to completely change your eating habits immediately. If you're already a healthy eater, great! However, I'd advise that you and your friends not to get involved in any diet trend or hype that seems to be taking over your social media and Facebook feeds. Another great illustration of how something that is intended to enhance your life turn into the source of your obsession, anxiety, stress and feelings of defeat. Marketing for supplements and nutrition are just as important as other forms of marketing. You shouldn't ever use the diet or nutrition program as the ultimate authority on nutrition. Make use of common sense avoid eating too much and try to eat more nutritious rather than junk. This is all you have to think about now. Do not embark on a low-carb diet now. There's something much more significant than that.

If you're thinking about what an eating plan that is healthier looks like, I'd recommend keeping a log of your food intake during the day for two or three consecutive days. Review the record. Does something stand out as risky? If, for instance, your eating pizza in frozen form or cookies at night and are feeling depressed there could be an excellent reason. We're not suggesting that you that you should eat salads and quinoa each day, but anyone could make one or two small adjustments to their daily eating routines and notice a huge improvement in their overall energy and mood. You can try to cut down on your intake of sugar and consume a few green foods each week. This is all you have to do to begin. Little steps, as with everything else, will help you progress to greater heights.

Exercise

Everyone's favorite exercise routine for your body and mind. Now, don't groan. Let's talk about it for a moment. There's no need to begin running for a marathon, or buy a full set of dumbbells to build your own home gym. I've already said it, and I'll repeat it for almost every suggestion in this list: one small step at one time. If you take things in small chunks and approach each step one at one time, you'll succeed more with your goals than when you attempt to do too much at once. It is essential when it comes to exercise to gauge your individual condition and abilities. Don't be comparing yourself to YouTube fitness stars who do crazy exercises every day and drinking shakes of protein. This is all about your personal development and improvement No one else's strategy will be as successful as yours.

Like the healthy eating habits the starting point is to look at what you're already doing and then move to the next intensity. That's all. If you're someone who loves exercising but is unable to find time to get it done and you're not getting enough time, I'm calling for you to come out! Training isn't about how long but rather how hard you're willing to work. I'm talking about only a few minutes a day to begin. If you're beginning with nothing the goal is to find ways to stand or walk instead of sitting. If you're able to, take in a stroll around the block or head to the park and walk around a bit. If you're at home take a break from your work and engage in a physical activity every couple of hours to make sure your blood circulation is pumping slightly more. The key is to make small changes. Change those little changes into habits, and focus on advancing to the next rung.

Many people think they require a costly gym membership in order to get in better in shape. It's not the case. There are a lot of exercises you can complete at home using no equipment or space that are great to boost your overall health. You might be a bit unique in that you're trying to be a competitor in bodybuilding competitions. However, most of us can notice a significant increase in energy, mood and overall health after simple converting some of your sitting time into some exercise. Look up the web or to YouTube for help if you're not sure of how to proceed. Squats as well as sit-ups and push-ups plansk holds, jogging running, walking and dancing do not require any apparatus and are performed virtually anywhere you'd like to do doing it. If you believe it could inspire you to do it with an accomplice take it! Join a fitness group class each week if you believe that it will be more enjoyable. The goal is to add a bit of physical exercise to your routine that is equal to more than what you've been doing prior to. Don't overburden yourself by attempting to begin an extreme 30-day challenge or 5 day workout routine. Your current focus is your mind. Don't get it cluttered with the same clutter you've spent so much effort to gain clarity.

Take time to take care of yourself regularly Another one that could mean a variety of things to individuals. The concept of making time for yourself could means setting aside time each day to do activities that make you feel relaxed and happy you. The only thing I'm going make is to do not make this a eating junk food or chocolate time. Chocolate can make you feel good...for only a couple of minutes...but all in all, it would be a horrible decision to develop the habit of eating junk food to make up for "you" moment. There are many other healthier options!

Do you like massages? Of course, the majority of people don't get daily massages however, maybe once or twice each month, you'll get an expert massage. Every day Find something that calms you, and then set aside one hour or more to do it. Even if it's just time to nap! Take a break, read a book, light candles, or take a break that calms your mind, and doesn't cause you to get up. This is about unwinding and not taking the pressure of the day with something noisy and distracting for the remainder time, the objective is to quiet your body and mind. Stretching is a fantastic option to accomplish this, particularly when you've been in your office chair for the entire day. Perhaps you'd like to talk with your partner or acquaintance over a cup of coffee. If you're in a position to do so think about it, you can brainstorm on the paper prior to selecting something that appeals to you.

To-do lists

A lot of us want to keep our day-to-day routines organized and that's wonderful. The issue with overthinking comes in when we be obsessed with getting every task on our list including those that aren't essential. A key part of creating good habits is understanding the right time to say no to things that you simply do not have the energy to accomplish if it's not essential. If you're feeling stressed, but you're working towards changing your lifestyle and habits and you're able to do so, then you'd rather not attend an outing for work or a birthday celebration with the friend of a person who you don't know well. If you feel that your time is better spending it at home, relaxing or doing something you love Then you should make a decision for yourself. There is no need to offer your energy and time to others only because they want it. Obligation is a major influence in many people's lives. A lot of people feel guiltiest when they fail to respond to solicitations or invitations. This is only another piece of clutter that is building within your head, leading to a lot of thinking. Thoughts of guilt and feelings are as potent as any other emotion and you need to protect yourself from them.

Make a list of your tasks according to the order of priority. It is obvious that grocery shopping for your children's meals comes prior to cutting the hedges in your front yard. This chore is a bit further down the list. Make a separate list of tasks you have to complete today as well as things you need to complete this week. This will allow your brain some space and ease. Instead of the list of 20 things you need to complete today, you could get to 5 or 6 tasks this morning and the remainder will be scheduled for later in the week based on your energy and time.

Get help whenever you require it.

This could be a huge problem for those who also are overachievers and perfectionists! Sometimes, we take on too much and we feel pressured to push ourselves over the edge to accomplish the things we've promised. Do not try to be a superman or superwoman. There will be instances when you require help particularly when you're trying to balance work and a household. Discuss the issue with your family members and your friends and you'll discover that the majority times they will be willing to assist you. It is crucial to not feel as if you are an insignificant person for seeking assistance. Nobody can go through life by themselves. This is your chance to build bonds and create new relationships while learning to work with one another. You'll feel more relaxed while your bonds grow stronger.

Be thankful

The process of clearing the mind and body of any clutter also involves cleansing your mind of negative emotions. Once you have begun to clear the negative thoughts and clutter in your head and also the clutter that are associated with negative emotions, it is crucial that you begin replacing the negative thoughts by positive thoughts. In the beginning, it might require some time and effort to keep you going however, eventually, the aim is to become automatic in your thoughts.

The power of gratitude is powerful to the brain. It is able to instantly transform an unhappy, stressful day into something hopeful and positive. Instead of dwelling on the problems you're confronted with and the things that you do not have, consider the many wonderful things that happen in your life you can be grateful for. Even the smallest things. Did you pay your utility bill each month? This is something you should be grateful for. Do you have people who love you and you enjoy spending time with? A lot of people don't. So be thankful. Are your beds nice and soft, with clean sheets? You can look forward to a relaxing night and be thankful. There are many reasons around you to feel thankful and it's important to notice them every day.

It's a time to be grateful. It's a time of lovely, warm emotions. It also helps you focus your attention on what's happening before you and surrounding you in the present moment. Many of us are distracted by thoughts of yesterday , or the week that preceded it, or years before...then our thoughts shift to the future and what's going on this weekend, and the next month and the year to come... Do you ever take a moment to look at your surroundings and feel grateful for the present moment in your life? This is so vital and I would like you to include this in your top priorities while you develop new positive lifestyle habits.

Chapter 17: How to Utilize Neuroplasticity to Reverse bad habits

It is possible to alter the bad habit? Are you able to replace restrictive practices with better practices?

This is the fact that many people believe is possible through Neuroplasticity.

What exactly is neuroplasticity? And what can it do to aid you in developing healthy habits?

Simply put, the concept of neuroplasticity is described as:

The way in which the cerebrum arranges itself through the process of framing new connections throughout the course of the course of

It's been suggested that the mind facilitates adaptation to exercises due to changing circumstances and changes in physical condition. Neuroplasticity allows your mind to be transformed by training and preparation.

Neuroplasticity could assist you in developing a daily Habit?

It's a common belief that when we are adulthood, we aren't able to change the habits that have developed over the course years of our life. We're told that nerve cells removed don't recover.

It's possible that this is true, but this doesn't stop the cerebrum from altering the way we do things. People can alter their behavior. The primary way you stop becoming a person is if you stop developing and learning.

What are the most frequent times you've heard about a grown-up who has returned back to school in order to acquire new information?

What are the most common instances of an older adult returning to learn a new exchange?

How can overweight people train their brains to become naive and athletic?

The possibilities for these changes are created through retraining your brain to think in a different manner. Neuroplasticity allows you to modify your thoughts to alter routines that are harmful to your daily life. It is possible to transform your concept into the kind of design you'd like your new habit to be.

Your mind is a vital asset. It can accomplish almost everything you can put your mind to. Therefore, if you must change your day to day habit, it will adapt to the new changes.

What can Neuroplasticity do to help you Remove Your Negative Habits

Bad habits: we all are all guilty of these. Whatever it is, whether it's that seems insignificant like gnawing the nails (liable) or something more authentic, like smoking cigarettes, everyone has at least one bad habit they'd like to get rid of.

The issue is that it's hard to carry out. If you've had several times of doing this in the past, whether you did it deliberately or not it's not very easy to wake up one day and think "all done, I'm done.'

But, it does not mean that getting out of an addiction is impossible. In reality, neuroleadership professional and author of the upcoming book , 'Footing' Kristen Hansen, says the most important factor is a basic process known as neuroplasticity.

In essence, neuroplasticity is the brain's ability to adapt and adapt. Through the process of forming new neural associations throughout life it is possible for the mind to'rearrange itself' and adapt to the changing needs of our society.

Self-guided Neuroplasticity is the ability to alter your personal mind. This is the method Hansen claims can assist in changing our behavior.

What are the negative effects of bad habits?

"Habits structures as easy ways for us to save our time or money or make us feel more comfortable," Hansen revealed to HuffPost Australia.

"So one of the models is If you're focused and take a bite of an ice cream cone is a way to feel good even in the midst of a bad moment. If you do it again, or three times it could become an habit.

"These alternative ways are designed as they are more established neural pathways. Furthermore, I'm not just talking about the massive habit of smoking cigarettes or drinking, but every and every habit could be something like getting caught up in the rest of your watch each day.

"Whenever it happens you're making it an habit."

What can I do to stop my bad habit?

167

1. Identify your habits

In the first place it is important to mention that not all habits need to be broken. In fact, there's an unbending idea as positive habits that need to be strengthened.

"The most important thing is to consider the extent to which activities we engage in in our lives have recently shifted towards becoming routines that aren't beneficial to the people we love," Hansen said.

"Huge quantities of our habits serve us. Therefore, if we exercise five times per week, it is an effective routine.

"I think the main goal is to figure out which areas of your daily life have habits that are beneficial to you and which ones don't to those which aren't working for you.

"Identifying them and notifying them is the first step."

2. Find out how to alter the cerebrum

As outlined by Hansen the author, it's not that easy to simply get rid of an habit. The most important thing is to substitute one habit for another.

"We must create fresh neural connections by being more vigilant," Hansen said. "If we pay conscious awareness of our reactions and how respond."

"When you begin to be aware of your triggers, then we'll be looking to participate as a substitute reaction" Hansen proceeded. "This is a 'better choice' reaction, our choice in contrast against the standard.

"The concept is to think of every time we feel the desire to change or improve the habit, to create an alternative habit that we're more attentive to. If you're in need of a sweet due to something else you're focusing on your work, you can turn on the kettle to enjoy a cup of tea."

3. Be aware of the goal

In order for you to stay on the right track, Hansen says it's essential to have a clear understanding of your goal.

"Ask yourself, not only "What do I want to accomplish and what date', but also "What would it look like, and how will I feel once I get there at my destination?' she stated.

169

"Bring the goal to life in your brain through imaginative representations and connecting to your emotions.

"For example, 'I'll be a non-smoker by December and I'll be a more healthy, fit and attractive person. I'll be more happy confident, happy and content'."

4. Concentrate on the new way we have to frame

We've now figured out how to replace your "bad" habit with a more positive habit, but Hansen states that it is essential to really put your energy into the new habit if you're hoping to keep it.

"Consideration can be defined in terms of the quantity and the quality of - that is how often and with what intensity we pay attention to things," she said.

"It's significant as neuroplasticity anticipates to be able to frame the new neural pathway to frame.

"We could put updates on our phone, engage in an instructor, or share our goal to our partner. These are amazing ways to create visit-based tokens of what we're trying to accomplish."

5. Make sure you give yourself positive feedback

Although this might sound a bit cliché, Hansen says it's a vital component of neuroplasticity.

"Reward yourself for the small achievements, rather than investing too much energy blaming ourselves for the areas we're not doing so well," she said.

"This positive feedback can cause us to feel better because it ends becoming a bit like a 'hit' to our cerebrums. When we say "good for you to ourselves or someone else says it dopamine gets released. Our minds become dependent. This is like giving ourselves a carrot, in a sense."

What is the length of time it will take to be able to come out of the grip of a habit?

"To how much it will take to establish a new habit depends on the person," Hansen said. "It is all about the amount of effort you put into it to develop the new habit and how much attention you give to the new method.

"However to be totally sincere, I've never seen anyone succeed on another behavior in less than three to one month.

"The most important thing is to be aware that we can reach a higher percentage in our capacity as individuals or as guardians, administrators, or co-conspirators if we become increasingly aware of the way we react to events and not always react in a controlled manner.

"Rather than simply trying to eliminate negative habits it's essential to be aware that we can develop many new habits to support us en our way.

It's an important part of getting the most out of our lives , and getting the most effective out from ourselves."

Chapter 18: Concentration and Concentration

One of the biggest challenges of navigating our neuroplasticity is our ability concentrate and focus. You may have a task right in front of you, yet you could be able to find it impossible to focus. This chapter we'll assist you in understanding the ways and reasons to concentrate.

How to focus can be difficult.

Accessing new information to study, as well as useful sources of information not the main issue. The issue in being a student is that it is extremely difficult to concentrate and focus. If you want to improve both of these there are a few actions you can take doing. The first is to ensure that you're checking for your general physical and mental wellbeing. Are you receiving the right diet, the correct quantity of physical exercise enough sleep and do you manage your anxiety?

These are the essential elements to ensure that you are at a high concentration and focus.

Sleep-deprived people will experience impaired cognitive functioning. If you're looking to be sure that you're giving yourself the capacity to focus on the things that matter. You must be in touch with everything. Apart from that there are other things that could cause a problem to concentrate.

If you are always distracted by your thoughts, then it can be hard to concentrate.

Perhaps you're worried and anxious about what you'll perform later in the day. You might be at the back of class , learning the details needed for a test however, you're that you're worried you're of having to be unable to pass the exam.

Maybe someone is trying to speak about you. However, you're concerned about making sure you're listening that you aren't able to hear any of their words. This may directly affect your ability to focus. It's challenging. However, if you begin to understand the reason you're not able to focus, it'll be much easier to figure out the solution to concentrate more effectively.

As we've already discussed, one of the main reasons it's the most difficult to concentrate is that you're not multitasking correctly.

There are times when it's hard to focus since you don't have a keen interest in what you're studying. In this section, we'll offer a couple of targeted exercises to do and also provide tips to help you to combat boredom and defeat the issue of prioritization. We will first dive deeper into multitasking.

Multitasking

The world is populated by numerous people with an interest or a passion that they would like to pursue. There are endless possibilities of what we can be done in the next few years. But, we won't be able to accomplish everything. This is the most difficult pill to take. Sometimes, there will to be certain things that you have to ignore and take care of what you have.

Have you ever been to vacation only to find that you didn't go to that place you'd like to visit or even discovered the location you'd like to go to and didn't get the chance? That's okay. Don't get stressed over the things you aren't able to accomplish. The most important thing is that we tackle every new challenge to conquer it with the best of our abilities. We've already talked about the necessity of not multitasking. However, let's examine some practical strategies you can employ to ensure that you stop doing this.

The first step is to remove your phone. This is difficult for some people to accomplish. It's like you are constantly receiving texts, emails, phone calls and the list goes on. Every time it happens you have the option of looking at the messages. Sometimes, this could make us feel stressed. What happens if something terrible happens? What happens if something goes wrong? If we have our phones in our hands and we get all the notifications, it could be distracting. Nowadays, phones are a necessity in our modern society. They aid us in our daily lives and remain connected. We can also learn new information by using numerous apps.

But they're also a major cause of disorientation. Make a few rules to yourself when using your phone. Set time frames throughout the day you can spend doing nothing but use your phone. If it's for 15 minutes, one hour, even two hours it's acceptable. Make sure to set aside this time to not sit in front of your mobile when you're doing that, it'll make it less appealing to glance on your smartphone for 5 or 10 minutes at a time during the course of your day. Put your phone in a different room. It's tempting to carry your phone around inside your purse or close to you throughout the day. If you're studying It's easy to reach out and take out your phone.

Place it in your kitchen cabinet or in a drawer in the bathroom or put it under your bed (just make sure you leave it there when you're asleep). Whatever you do, you must remove yourself from your mobile to ensure that you don't get likely to be enticed to glance at it. You must get out of the habit of checking it at the same time each day. Some individuals do it first at the beginning of their day, and it is the final thing they do before going to going to bed. A few people do it while sitting at their table eating dinner. Some will do it when they're at the restroom. No matter what, you will take note of the patterns of using your smartphone and breaking the habit.

Smartphones aren't a problem often. They're not the cause of the problems we must fight. They can be a wonderful source of education. It is possible to download ebooks, you can surf through the internet or play games. Whatever you'd like do will most likely perform it using your smartphone. But, if we're not vigilant, it can turn out to be harmful, it could affect our lives, and could cause harm. Move your phone to a different place. Make a change, identify patterns and make use of it to benefit yourself, not to serve as a source of distraction or to ease boredom. Then, when you're multitasking, ensure you become conscious of how much focus you're paying to essential tasks. If you are asked to perform something that you aren't sure you can accomplish, you must learn to tell them no. This is one of the toughest tasks for people to master. If you don't say yes to someone, they might not be asking for some thing again in the near future. Who knows if that means you are missing opportunities. Do not be a victim of this thought. If you're always worried of what might result if you refuse to say then you'll always say yes. It's not a one-size-fits-all-thing. You have the option of saying"no. Sometimes, you'll have to affirm yourself, other times, you should do what's most beneficial for you. You shouldn't cause harm to others. Be aware of this especially if you know someone else who wouldn't be able to do the same thing for you.

If you're not sure and then you observe that people have left your life, but they're not in a state of being present, perhaps that's an indication that they shouldn't be around at all in the first instance.

If you are forced to begin making use of external sources to keep your from multitasking One method that is secure is to have an iPhone or any other device that requires a password try entering it wrongly multiple times. If you enter it incorrectly enough, it could keep you locked out for between a minute and an hour or whatever it takes, based on the kind of phone you have. This is a good way to ensure that the moment you get your phone back and try to use it, you will not be in a position to use it. You can also switch your phone into airplane mode for the time you're in need of. There are other applications that stop certain websites from certain time periods for your laptop. Use these strategies to avoid being distracted and multitasking as often as you can.

Accelerated Learning

There's a lot of information available to discover, it's important to know how you can speed up your learning and get the greatest results. Accelerated learning is the method of absorbing new information at an accelerated rate. Although it may seem like this could be a result in you not retaining as much information however, it's an effective method of understanding the basics of learning and to understand smaller specifics.

Let's begin by understanding the ways you can read faster. It will be necessary to go through the books you're planning to be learning to understand what you're likely to read. Of of course, if you're to be reading a novel book, it could lead to spoiling the ending or other important plot elements which is why it should only be used with non-fiction books you're studying.

The first thing you'll want to do is read through each chapter, and then break them down and examine subheadings, too. Be attentive to the tables of content and connect the dots before you start reading to make it easier to understand concepts as you read through the text. Additionally ensure that you've identified the keywords you'll want to search for. For instance, if you're taking a test in the book you're reading next week and the book has the words that must be understood or important points, these are the resources of what you'll be looking out for as you read through the book.

The next thing you need to do is to begin your reading. One way to speed up your reading is to focus on the first sentence of each paragraph in a single reading. Then, you can skim through the rest part of your paragraph. It's because the primary purpose of the paragraph needs to be outlined from the beginning. The rest of the paragraph will be the description, and then more supporting information to reinforce the concept.

You could also concentrate on reading the final sentence, as it will help to speed things to flow into another paragraph. When you read it, you'll also need to work on reducing the subvocalization. This it's the voice that's at the behind of your head that interprets what you read as. What you need to be able to do is silence this voice to read more quickly. Sometimes, you become distracted by your words and stumble over what you're trying to convey because you're focused on struggling to say the word you're reading.

Conclusion

Next step would be getting to use the mental models to meet our personal requirements. There are many kinds of mental models and we attempted to go through the most efficient ones and those that can aid you in making choices, plan the time you have, as well as accomplish your goals. Once you have the structure in place that your mental model can offer it will be apparent that it's simpler to attain the results you desire. Your mind will be more at liberty to think in a creative manner instead of focusing on things that aren't really important to you.

This book took some time to explore the various mental models at your disposal. We talked about the things the mental model is about, the most powerful mental models that are able to be beneficial to you, as well as these mental models, and their ability to function with various circumstances that you face in your life. This can allow us to be aware of all the different aspects that they bring and ensure that we're employing them in the appropriate scenarios.

www.ingramcontent.com/pod-product-compliance
Lightning Source LLC
Chambersburg PA
CBHW060330030426
42336CB00011B/1283